GAPS Stories

Personal Accounts of Improvement and
Recovery through the GAPS Nutritional
Protocol

Compiled by

Medinform Publishing

Medinform

© Medinform Publishing, 2012

GAPS Stories

ISBN 10: 978-0-9548520-5-2
ISBN 13: 978-0-9548520-5-4

First published in the United Kingdom in 2012 by
Medinform Publishing

The right of Medinform Publishing to be identified as the author and publisher of this work has been asserted by them in accordance with the Copyright, Patent and Designs Act 1988.

"Gut and Psychology Syndrome™" and "GAPS™" are international trademarks of Dr Natasha Campbell-McBride and their use is strictly prohibited withourt prior written permission from Dr Natasha Campbell-McBride.

Typeset by Cambrian Typesetters, Frimley, Surrey

Contents

The stories are grouped roughly according to health conditions. However, as every person has more than one health problem, there is a lot of overlap. Please, refer to the Index at the end of the book if you are interested to read about a particular health problem or a particular symptom. Reference should also be made to the book Gut And Psychology Syndrome and the website www.gaps.me.

Introduction   vii

FAMILIES

1. **Kitty Ingham**   3

2. **Linda Paterson**   9

3. **Anna Breheney**   18

4. **Ophelia**   24

5. **Brenda Scott**   41

6. **Nichole Sawatzky**   46

7. **K.H.**   49

8. **Nancy**   52

9. **Melinda DeGier**   55

10. **Cara Comini**   58

11. **Kris Gustafson**   61

12. **Denise**   67

13. **Dawn Wiley**   76

14. **Sonia Zukoski**   79

15. **Lynne M. George**   82

16. **Susanna**   84

17. **Susan White**   90

18. **Eileen**   95

19. **Kim Schuette**   100

20. **Kathleen Mills**   107

21. **Gabriela Mikova**   115

22. **J.F.**   120

23. **M.C.**   125

24. **Anne**   127

25. **Jeni**   135

26. **J.B.**   149

ADULTS

1. A.   157

2. Tara   161

3. Ashley R. Hathaway   166

4. Shann Jones   169

5. A.S.   172

6. Aaron Falbel   175

7. Janice   181

8. Hella D.   183

9. Gerald   189

10. John   196

11. Lydia Rose   199

12. Kathleen Bush   206

13. S.K. Smith   211

14. Anonymous   216

15. R. Fiano   217

16. Starlene D. Stewart   220

17. Gawain Hammond   224

18. Emily Jane Williams   227

19. **Sherry Miller** 229

20. **Catherine Cruchon** 232

21. **Marijke de Jong** 244

22. **D.** 247

23. **Emily Jane Butler** 252

24. **Michelle** 256

25. **Maria** 259

Introduction

GAPS stands for Gut And Psychology Syndrome and Gut And Physiology Syndrome. I have created this term in 2004 to describe the plethora of health problems which stem from an unhealthy gut. Recent research has demonstrated that about 90% of all cells and genetic material in the human body is gut flora – a very complex mass of microbes residing in your digestive system. In a healthy person this microscopic world is dominated by beneficial species of microbes, which work in harmony with your body, making sure that you are well-nourished, protected from pathogens and toxins, and that your immune system is healthy and robust. In a GAPS person the gut flora is unhealthy – it is dominated by pathogenic microbes. As a result the person develops multiple health problems. The GAPS Nutritional Protocol has been designed to bring your gut flora back to normal, heal your digestive system and remove all the health problems related to this condition. To get a full understanding of GAPS please read my book *Gut And Psychology Syndrome*.

Since developing the GAPS Nutritional Protocol I have been receiving letters from GAPS people from all over the world. It is an honour and a privilege for me to publish these letters! These stories were written by real people, who have overcome their real health problems. Every one of these people feels that they have learned very valuable lessons on their healing journey: lessons which they are keen to pass to others, who may be struggling through the same difficulties. Please, use these stories as case studies, to study how to progress through your personal healing, and how to deal with problems that you may have to face on the way.

There is nothing more valuable than real life experience! When you have lived through something, fought the battle and won, you know what is true and what is false, what works and what doesn't. You don't need 'scientific evidence' or 'expert opinion' to tell you; and if they dare to tell you otherwise, you know that they simply don't know what they are talking about... Because you possess the truth, you have lived it and you have earned it the hard way!

Many of these stories are humbling: the kinds of horrific problems that people have had to deal with are hard to imagine for the majority of us. Yet, these wonderful people tell their stories with such humour and such grace!

I would like to thank every one of these people for sharing their very personal stories with the world! This is an act of selfless benevolence, born out of the desire to help others, without asking for anything in return. Thank you!

Dr Natasha Campbell-McBride
Author of Gut and Psychology Syndrome

FAMILIES

1

Kitty Ingham

Key words: reflux, food allergies, immune system insufficiency, Kawasaki disease, chronic constipation, digestive problems

My son was born in March 2000 in the Mathilda Hospital in Hong Kong, by natural delivery but with an epidural. Looking back he was not as healthy as I then thought he was. His stomach was swollen and he cried a lot. He didn't sleep well and he didn't have a healthy complexion. We left the hospital after three days thinking that I had a healthy baby boy, but my son and I were both admitted to hospital when my son was one month old, as we were both suffering from exhaustion.

In the hospital my son was diagnosed as having suspected reflux and put on Zantac and other adult drugs. The doctor told me I had to put him in a baby car seat so his food would stay down in his stomach and not come back up. I did this but I was not comfortable with it at all. How could he digest his food by being folded up double in a car seat all day whilst consuming heavy adult drugs?

After two months I put my son on formula and this way at least I regained my strength. I was given *The Contented Little Baby Book* by Gina Ford, which brought a well-needed consistent schedule to my daily and nightly routine which worked very well for my son and me.

When my son was eight months old his cheeks were red raw and bleeding for several months. By then I had introduced him to quite a few new foods including baby rice, meat, vegetables and fruit. As I thought that the bleeding cheeks had something to do with food allergies I reintroduced all his food again in rotation and removed chicken and mango after which his skin cleared up.

My son did not have the MMR in one cocktail, but separately. Just after he received his measles injection things started to get worse. He

3

became extremely constipated. He would make himself vomit to push out his stool. He also stopped drinking. He was admitted to hospital with severe dehydration and very high temperature and put on a drip for three days during which he improved rapidly.

The many doctors we saw for my son's constipation problem prescribed various drugs but none of them worked. They only seemed to make it worse. I tried all the diet interventions with orange juice first thing in the morning, fibre solutions, lots of prunes added to his diet but nothing worked. He was on 30 ml of Dufalex a day but no stool would come out. When another doctor saw my son regarding his extreme constipation problems, he told us that it was my son's reaction to me and my husband and that he was intentionally playing up, because he (the doctor) had never seen a child not having a stool movement after so many drugs. He referred us to a child psychologist. By this stage my son had been in severe pain for over a year and looked dreadful. His stool was being cleared out by Microlax enemas every four to five days.

After explaining everything to the child psychologist, he told us that he had never seen this extreme behaviour in children as young as my son and seriously doubted that there were any psychological or reactive behavioural problems. The child psychologist could not give us any other advice than find a doctor who can identify the problem and consider going to Harley Street in London.

By this stage my son was three years old. He would still vomit trying to push out his stool unsuccessfully and we still had to use child enemas. He started to produce small 'pebble' stools in his underpants up to 20 times a day. His bottom became infected and the skin was cracked. He was in a lot of pain. Clearing your child out with Microlax is so distressing for child and parent alike.

My son's health was deteriorating. He had ear infection after ear infection. Because of this he would have many courses of antibiotics. He also developed asthma and bronchitis and was on different inhalers for his symptoms.

When my son contracted the chickenpox because of his weak immune system he had the worst case my GP had ever seen. His whole body was inflamed and his beautiful face was completely swollen. He had the spots for weeks on end and it took months before he was able to function normally again. He was tired and lethargic, and had purple rings under his eyes. If we went out over the weekend to see some friends and their children, my son would catch any bug going around and he had to stay in the following weeks to recover. We had registered my son for a private kindergarten and out of the nine months, he attended only two months.

Around this time my son started to develop uncontrollable tantrums. He also had many accidents. I found the accidents strange. Why would he fall over and always end up with a big head wound and stitches? He wasn't clumsy. Why did he always fall onto something hard and sharp when other children would sort of bounce back up. My son fell with his head against a radiator at my parents' house and ended up with 15 stitches just in his hairline on his forehead. Three months later he fell again on the corner of the climbing frame and ended up with seven stitches just about the eye. A week later he fell over at a friend's house and his whole mouth was bleeding. I was terrified and everywhere we went I could see the sharp corners or the other children pushing him which made him fall over again. Due to his poor immune system his skin wouldn't heal as quickly as it should have leaving big scars.

I started to think about the connection with his accidents and the food he had eaten beforehand. I went back to my GP for an allergy test. We did the *Elisa Blood Test* that was sent to the USA. The results came back with positive for IgG anti-gliadin (gluten) antibodies 98 units, which is very high. My son started his gluten-free diet in August 2003. I saw an improvement in his health but he was still very constipated. As the gluten-free diet is not easy to follow in Hong Kong, where it is not that common (yet) I came into contact with some autism websites where parents of autistic children start seeing improvement by combining a gluten-free diet with a casein-free diet for their children. I started to educate myself about the digestive system of my son. There was so much information out there (internet) which made lots of sense to me, so I also removed all dairy (casein) from my son's diet and saw further improvement. His mood improved, the ear infections disappeared and his asthma and bronchitis stopped.

Being on a gluten-and-casein-free diet improved his health but he was still quite a sickly child. He was still constipated although he now had some bowel movements by himself. But he developed many cases of conjunctivitis, impetigo and other skin infections. These would take weeks to clear up with the application of various dressings and ointments numerous times each day.

Then in May 2004 my son was diagnosed by our GP with Kawasaki disease. Kawasaki disease is an inflammation of the blood vessels. The most important blood vessels involved are those of the heart, including the coronary arteries. Kawasaki disease has become the most common cause of heart disease in children born without birth defects. If Kawasaki disease is not recognized and appropriately treated within 10 days, the risk of permanent damage increases. Children can die from the blood clots which form in the reserves where the blood vessels swell. Our GP referred us to a specialist in Hong Kong. We were too late for the initial treatment that can avoid the main symptoms. However, the specialist wanted to give my son an MRI scan. This involved injecting some solution into his veins, but the specialist could not tell us what was in it. It didn't make sense to me to give my son this scan which would probably scare him even more and would not change anything, as the only treatment known (after the initial stage) was aspirin. My son didn't have the scan. I called the Kawasaki helpline in the UK who were very helpful and I spent hours being comforted by the lady running the helpline. She got me in contact with a Kawasaki specialist in the UK who advised us on low doses of aspirin. The illness lasted for three whole months. During this time my son looked awful, often described for Kawasaki disease as looking like a panda; very pale with big black circles around his eyes. He received regular heart scans from the consultant in Hong Kong who was very helpful, looking to see if the arteries around the heart were swollen. He gave my son all the time needed to determine if he had permanent damage, which luckily he did not. Through this I learnt about the chemicals in paint, carpets, furniture, curtains and mattresses, and how my son's condition meant that he could not cope with them because he could not at that stage detoxify his body naturally. This is what I believed made him ill with Kawasaki disease.

I was still educating myself about the constipation and gut issues my son seemed to have. I was also trying to bake gluten-and-casein-free bread and tried to replace all my convenience food and snacks with gluten-and-casein-free ones. But there was more. He obviously had a very poor immune system and I didn't see more improvement in his health. Somebody mentioned to me about a diet that originated in the US by a doctor called Dr Haas. It was the ultimate gut healing diet as it was based on only mono-saccharides and this way the gut could heal itself. I strongly believed that it was my son's birthright to have the best chance in life (and for me that meant a healthy body); I was determined to learn everything I possibly could to make this happen for him. After educating myself about this diet I felt that my son had the best chance to get as close as possible to a healthy body with the diet invented by Dr Haas and improved by Dr Natasha Campbell-McBride.

I have had many telephone appointments with Dr Campbell-McBride, as I was very scared about taking my son's health in my own hands. I was also scared about not following the advice of specialists in Hong Kong, who wanted to remove part of his colon. I strongly believed that removing part of his gut would not take away the problem. Speaking to Dr Campbell-McBride I knew I was doing the right thing for my son. I was so relieved that I had found a doctor who was thinking with me, supporting me and my family through this and explaining how to go further with the diet.

For me the GAPS Diet was not so easy to follow. I found it very hard, particularly in the beginning. But my strong belief in the diet made me able to follow it for three full years. We started the GAPS Diet while still living in Hong Kong; during these three years we moved to the UK and are now living in Holland.

The GAPS Diet wasn't easy, but NOW FOR ME MIRACLES DO EXIST! I have seen with my own eyes that my very sickly child has improved in body and mind beyond my imagination! Before the diet, while living in Hong Kong, when I called my GP to make an appointment for my son, I was always allowed to get to his office straight away without waiting and be able to skip the queue. That was how sick my child was! My son is 11 years old now and I have not been to a doctor since the end of the first year after starting the diet! He is a healthy and happy boy!

I have learned an awful lot about what food and drink can do to your body and mind! With all the hard work it took I am now a lot wiser than I would have ever been without my son's health problems.

Sometimes, when I see parents with children in poor health I like to tell them about the diet. But unfortunately a lot of people do not go down that road for their own reasons. That does make me realize again that I have done something very special for my son, which I am very proud of.

Kitty Ingham has trained as a Certified GAPS Practitioner in 2012.

A comment from Dr Natasha

Thank you, Kitty, for your story! You are absolutely correct: our children deserve the best chance in life; it is their birthright! Being susceptible to every virus and bacteria going around is not normal. Suffering from chronic digestive problems is not normal. Being miserable, clingy and unable to cope with life is not normal. But so many parents are led to believe that their child should just 'cope' with poor health and poor quality of life; that there is 'nothing they can do'. Parents like Kitty, who do not accept this dogma, give their child the best option to live a happy and fulfilling life.

2

Linda Paterson

Key words: autism, fussy eating habits

My son's healing journey from autism

I live in Brisbane Australia and am a mother of Reilly diagnosed with autism at the age of three. We, parents, first identified our son's condition at age two, when his language had regressed and he stopped eating all my home-made meals, limiting his food intake to only a few items. Soon after this came self-harming behaviour when he would scratch his face, bite his arms and bang his head on the floor, causing scratch marks on his cheeks, bite marks on his arms and hands, and bruises on his forehead.

At two months of age and onwards his sleep was very abnormal and continued to worsen. He was awake every hour on the hour and there was nothing we could do to console him. All we could do was to place him in bed between us, but if we were to touch him he would scream. I had experienced this sort or avoidant-touch behaviour before in my work with disabled children. I expressed the idea of autism to my husband, but we quickly dismissed it as an overreaction, due to the lack of any other symptoms of autism.

I cringe now when I recall how we succumbed to the pressure of our son's paediatrician, who had surprised us with his abrupt advice to vaccinate our son with an additional meningococcal C vaccine at six weeks of age, followed by two boosters at 10 and 14 weeks of age. This vaccine is not advised on the Australian immunization program schedule until the age of 12 months, but our paediatrician created a fear in us with his fist in hand statement about life-threatening risk of contracting meningococcal infection before the age of 12 months. As a result our son received 3 additional vaccinations at a very young age,

9

when his immune system could simply not cope with them. I didn't know at the time that this vaccine only covered three out of 13 of the meningococcal C diseases, it did not cover many other types of meningococcal diseases, and according to the Australian Vaccination Network, the overall risk of death from meningococcal disease was extremely low – recorded at 1:000,000. Since then we also learnt that doctors are paid by pharmaceutical companies for the percentage of children they vaccinate.

Later we learned that about 50% of the vaccine ingredients was an aluminium adjuvant. Yes, it is hard to believe that almost 50% of every vaccine, we inject into our children, consist of this toxic metal. When our son was tested for exposure to toxic chemicals, it was aluminium poisoning that was revealed as the most alarming concern – it scored the highest above all other toxins in his body. The vaccines may not have been the cause of his autism, but, due to our son's weak immune system from birth, the vaccinations resulted in a direct insult on his immune system. Vaccines overloaded his body with toxins that his young detoxification system could not cope with. As his body struggled to detoxify, the toxic metals began to cause damage and symptoms had built up over time.

Having worked with disabled children before has prepared me well in applying my skills to helping my son. However, there is nothing that can prepare a parent for a child who displays behaviours that appear to show you: they do not want your love or affection. When your own child does not know your name or pushes your face away, won't let you console him when he is upset, bangs his head on the floor, bites himself and claws at his face, a mother feels helpless and depleted. This is what we lived with before we found what we needed to heal our son.

Since then I have watched Reilly transform rapidly from being in a world of his own, with no communication and self-harming behaviours, to an interactive five-year-old boy gaining quickly on his peers in the areas of social and developmental progress. Apart from early home intervention programmes, run by myself, coupled with speech therapy and support from his fully certified assistance dog, the only change I have made is the implementation of a strict GAPS Nutritional Protocol, inclusive of the GAPS Introduction Diet.

Arriving at that wonderful stage in Reilly's life was overwhelming and very rewarding! However it was not achieved without its challenges. Initially it took great leaps and bounds to get a diagnosis for Reilly, and this was followed by the search for treatment options. These options often take parents on a journey that requires a detailed map in order to find the right treatment. Parents of autistic children are familiar with this path: numerous conflicting options are time-consuming for parents to navigate: chelation therapy, stool analysis tests, hair analysis tests, IgG and IgE tests, an ever-increasing amount of supplements, confusing contradictions between doctors and other integrative therapists, not to mention the variety of diets. Is it gluten-free, casein-free, food elimination rotation diets, the Feingold diet, low phenols, body ecology diet, SCD, low oxalate diet or Nourishing Traditions? The list goes on, and one particular conference I attended even promoted a vegetarian diet for treating autism, outlining how bad consumption of meat and fats is. The choices are exhaustive, and making the right decision is paramount.

I took my son to several dieticians, health professionals and biomedical doctors to seek the best advice on diet and treatment for ASD. However, no direction or guidance on GAPS was offered, and collective advice conflicted with each other. Searching for the right treatment took a great deal of time, effort and money, with an ever increasing accumulation of new books. My academic research ability and knowledge, gained through my health science degree, coupled with my work in the disability and mental health field with the Department of Justice, was a valuable resource to me during that time. It was my own extensive research (involving travel to several destinations, including flights out of state to attend autism expos and a variety of conferences, seminars, workshops and presentations), that led me to the discovery of a little yellow book tucked in the corner at a Sydney Autism Expo. This yellow book became my bible – *The Gut and Psychology Syndrome* by Natasha Campbell-McBride.

Prior to GAPS my son was an extremely fussy eater, self-limiting his food range to an extreme minimum, resulting in a variety of deficiencies and nutritional problems. After two weeks on the Introduction Diet, he was eating everything we gave him and even asked for seconds. We would never have believed this possible if we had not seen it with our own eyes! The circles around his eyes were gone, he had gained weight, but more importantly, he was participating in lengthy conversations, socialising in ways never seen before, showing lots of affection and sharing his emotions. The list of improvements went on, but the rest of this story is yet to be revealed, as I believe my son will continue to heal and gain developmental ground with his peers, as he continues to progress with the GAPS Diet.

It would have been invaluable to have someone to show me how to make sauerkraut, homemade yoghurt, meat stocks and how to select the right cookware and storage containers. I won't lie, there was a time when I felt I lived in the kitchen and cried to the Gods in Heaven to help me with my struggles! But, as I became more confident in the kitchen, I found my passion and love for nourishing food. This does not mean that I am a great cook because I can still cook a hungry man's dinner, but now I know what to cook and how to prepare for it and, more importantly, why I am cooking it. My kitchen became the hub of my home; it is where I stir up my pot of love.

My biggest need for support and guidance was when my son had experienced severe 'die-off' reactions. It could have been very easy to stop and give up with the Intro Diet because my son had reacted severely to the release of toxins in his body. This was when my idea emerged to become a Nutrition Consultant for GAPS; I knew there had to be parents out their like me who needed this level of support. Since then Dr Natasha has trained hundreds of practitioners (including myself) across the globe, and many families now have the opportunity to get the support and guidance they need for their healing journey.

Fussy eating

GAPS is so powerful! I have referred so many people to the diet already and have had several parents over for tea to discuss and learn about the diet. Many parents ask the same question: *My child is a fussy eater and self-limits his diet. How am I going to get him to eat the GAPS food?* This was my number one question too. I sought answers everywhere, including standing up at seminars and asking several experts how this could be achieved.

Reilly's fussy eating was an understatement: he had extreme food aversions and oral sensory issues. He would only eat five foods, so we gave him the GAPS alternatives to what he liked, like crumbed chicken nuggets with almond meal, cooked in lard. Big mistake! He ate it, but it was by no means providing him with healing foods. All it did was eliminate the offending foods he needed to avoid and provide him with self-limiting alternatives. He did have withdrawals from dairy and grains and seemed to do much better without them, but he was just plugging along with his fussy little eating habits and made very little progress.

It was not until I decided to implement strict Applied Behaviour Analysis (ABA) strategies (explained in the GAPS book under the chapter 'It's feeding time! Oh, no!') that we saw an amazing change. We had to get him to eat the things his little body desperately needed. I thought: if I was going to do this, I needed to commit 100% and be well prepared, firm and consistent with my approach. The other key factor was to not give in to him and avoid giving him any other food, if he refused to eat what we offered. ABA needed to be planned with realistic goals and highly motivating rewards (motivating for Reilly!). We strategically designed some intervention tools tailored to his needs, that we knew he could work with and enjoy. With the use of the tools and ABA strategies we started to introduce new foods from the GAPS Introduction Diet.

All we gave him for two weeks was home-made soup and meat stock. This was very difficult: he gagged, screamed, self-harmed and vomited. When he learnt that he could get a reward (that he really desired), he complied with our requests. We worked as a husband-wife team together in the first few days in doing this. After a few days he began to detox and got sick, with some symptoms getting worse. He even went off eating his food altogether, which we later learnt was common at this stage. Although this was worrying, we nursed him through the detox stage as if it was a bad virus or flu, and gradually continued with giving him his soup and stock in small amounts. By the middle of the second week, he asked for seconds, and then thirds, and we thought 'hey ho, stop, your belly is full now'. He actually wanted and desired the food that he completely struggled with only 10 days ago, and wanted lots of it!

On the second week we started him on stage two of the GAPS Intro Diet with lamb casserole and vegetables. We got all the ABA tools and items out ready to go through it again, but to our amazement he ate it and was really enjoying it without any ABA intervention. He then wanted to eat bananas and other fruits, and foods that we could never get him to eat before. I did not think he would eat the banana, so I gave it to him and, to my surprise, he ate it and asked for another, and then asked for an apple. Unfortunately we could not give him the second banana or any other fruit, because we wanted to stick to the intervention plan.

I never would have believed it if I had not seen it with my own eyes! It was at this point that I said to my husband "parents need to know this!" So here I am telling people: IT IS POSSIBLE TO GET RID OF FUSSY EATING IN A CHILD! And the parents CAN do what seems impossible to achieve! As a result, I have had the pleasure of watching many other committed parents, who thought it was not possible, see their own little fussy eaters transform in 10 days.

If all it takes is 100% commitment from parents, good healing food, an individual ABA plan with a few dollars spent on some very moti-vating rewards, then it is well worth it! I would have paid hundreds just to have someone get him to eat some nourishing foods! But instead we did it ourselves, and all the money went into our son with his rewards. If you think that you can do it, then I strongly support your success, as I have seen others achieve it, who thought it was not possible. *There is something about the healing properties in the meat stock and soup that begins to repair the microvilli and enterocytes in the gut wall, which consequently interrelate with the mind, taste and adjustment of sensory issues with food.* GAPS somehow changes all this, so it is well worth the effort to give it a go.

I know, breaking fussy eating habits can be more difficult with older children, but where there is a will there is a way. Just keep talking to your child and educating them if you can. You know your child better than anyone else, so you will know what will best motivate him/her, and what strategies to use in implementing an ABA plan. Remember, the best desired outcome for fussy eaters is achieved by combining ABA with the implementation of the GAPS Introduction Diet. Have faith, give it all you have and think of food as your love! What do you have to lose?

Thanks to all our efforts by the age of five Reilly started Prep in a mainstream school, where he transitioned nicely and joined a soccer team on weekends. He developed hobbies and interests in computers and sports, and he was reading books two to three years ahead of his peers. No more self-harming behaviours or screaming tantrums on the floor. He became a very affectionate little boy loved by all and who loved to interact with his peers. Although his speech development was only slightly behind his peers, we had confidence that he would catch up in good time as he continued progressing with the GAPS Protocol.

Supportive families make for an easier transition in implementing the GAPS Protocol. I know this first hand as my husband has supported GAPS; he participates in many of the cooking activities and fermentation of food. We often called ourselves the octopus team in the morning. One was juicing whilst the other was preparing lunches and cooking up some breakfast.

It is also very important to include your children in the education process on good nutrition and cooking in the kitchen. Our son drags a chair to the kitchen every time he hears the kitchen utensils clanging together. He gets his tasting and mixing spoon ready and loves to juice and crack a perfect egg every morning. Our daughter submitted a video to A Current Affair for the Top Mini Chef Competition with her brother as an assistant in cooking GAPS recipes. Her application of cooking skills was aired every night on A Current Affair for a week, until my daughter was awarded as a finalist and was flown to Sydney to compete with the final eight contestants. She did very well in winning many kitchen appliances and cookware, all of which found a nice home in our kitchen.

I have devoted the GAPS Australia Website to both Dr Natasha and Peter Campbell-McBride who know too well what it is like to work as a team in implementing the GAPS Protocol and the importance of supporting one another during the process. I know I speak for hundreds of families when I say that we are grateful to Dr Natasha for pioneering this programme and teaching us how to do it for ourselves. Dr Natasha has shown us with the many stories she has collected since the launch of her first book that, with the right level of support and commitment, it is possible to turn your health around!

Today

Reilly is now seven and a half in grade two (mainstream school) and has caught up with his peers in areas of communication and comprehension. He continues to be a confident reader ahead of his years and obtains high standards in all academic subjects. He enjoys learning music and playing guitar, he has recently joined a rugby team and contributes to scoring a try in almost every game. New people we meet are unaware of his initial diagnosis of autism, and we are as proud as punch with his delightful personality. Of course there are some slight differences that we are aware of ourselves which are unique to Reilly, but he would not be the same little boy without them and we cherish these endearing mannerisms. He continues to eat everything we put in front of him and remains on the GAPS diet with his favourite food being pork fat and crackle. He remains on the GAPS diet as it provides him with all the nourishing food he needs, and we find it easy enough to maintain. He has recently enjoyed the rare meal at a restaurant and tolerates the meals well. We do select restaurant meals that are more in-line with the GAPS diet, but it is reassuring to know that his gut has healed to allow him to digest and tolerate foods outside of the home. Our next adventure is to embark on a short holiday without taking an esky of food with us. Perhaps we will just take some easy simple snacks with us for our first trip.

Thank you Dr Natasha for bringing our son back to us and may God Bless you for every angel you return.

Linda Paterson runs a company called GAPS Australia, giving support to families on the GAPS Programme.

A comment from Dr Natasha

Another autistic child recovered! Reilly is leading a normal happy life, as any boy of his age should, thanks to his parent's dedication.

Linda' experience with fussy eating is extremely valuable! Fussy eating habits in autistic and other GAPS children are very common. It is the first hurdle parents have to overcome in order to implement any diet. And indeed, many parents don't believe at the beginning that it is even possible to overcome this hurdle. Yet, as Linda has observed, family after family do it and never turn back. Your child is fussy with food for very solid physiological reasons and not because he or she is 'naughty'. GAPS Introduction Diet changes the physiology in the gut and the brain, allowing the child to start perceiving food appropriately. As a result, fussy eating becomes history, which is soon forgotten. And indeed it can happen in just 10 days! Thank you, Linda, for this wonderful and very motivating story!

3

Anna Breheney

Key words: autism, fussy eating

Greek Grandmother Power

From the moment I read Dr Natasha's personal testimony of how she helped her son to recover from autism, there was never a doubt in my mind that I would implement the GAPS Diet in our house for my son, aged four, diagnosed with autism.

I read Dr Natasha's book, made soup, sauerkraut, ghee, yogurt and lard. All the while my heart trembled with fear – not because of the massive job I knew I was about to undertake, nor because of how difficult I imagined it would undoubtedly be, nor even because of the scary thought that perhaps it wouldn't work – but because of the seemingly impossible task of how on earth I was going to get my son to eat this soup and broth, let alone sauerkraut and all the other unusual stuff!

James had limited his diet severely to a minute variety of sweet and starchy foods and processed carbohydrates. And even these did not interest him too much. I certainly couldn't get him interested in any food enough to actually want to feed himself. Instead, I would follow him around the house to try to get in a mouthful of rice here, a bit of pasta there, a GF cookie or glass of rice milk. Often I would feed him in the bathtub as this was the only place I could contain him. So my major fear and concern was how on earth I was going to get him to eat GAPS food!

I had consulted with Linda Peterson at GAPS Australia and she had given me strategies and advice, which were very helpful in preparing me mentally and giving me hope that this really could be done. Hearing her own personal testimony about her son was also very helpful, because I thought, hey, this is real, it actually does happen, so maybe, just maybe, it could happen for us.

The one thing Linda said which stood out to me was that we had to get large quantities of this food into James and the more he ate the more he would heal and the quicker the healing would happen, so we began, with this thought foremost in my mind.

I had my mum all prepared. She very kindly offered to come and help me every day and has actually kept coming even now as we begin week six, and I suspect she will keep coming until I just don't need her to come any more. My mum and dad adore James and would do absolutely anything to help him heal and see a better life ahead for him than we had thus far been given hope for.

So I worded her up. I explained ABA strategies to a 70-year-old woman brought up in a village in Greece. Little did I know that my mum was to give *me* a few lessons of her own, by bringing a whole new dimension to our GAPS introduction – she was to be our secret weapon!

We have another son, Thomas, a typically developing child who is aged two and was also going on the diet, just because it was easier to have them both doing it. Because James adores Yaya (my mum) as much as she adores him, he insisted she was to be the one to feed him, so I would concentrate on Thomas and mum on James.

What a nightmare! They both refused to eat the first day. Second day Tom ate but not James. Third day James began to have a little teaspoon of broth at a time, with the promise of a tiny bit of coconut oil with Manuka honey for a reward.

By this time they were both starving. They were like druggies on withdrawal, whining and crying all day, pining for all the foods they could no longer have, searching the now empty pantry and fridge for anything and being utterly miserable that first week. It was excruciating. But as the days passed, Yaya wooed James into eating. I watched her in amazement out of the corner of my eye while feeding Tom, who was nowhere near as difficult to handle. She used the art of distraction skillfully. She would hold the spoon before his mouth while simultaneously talking calmly yet enthusiastically. She told him stories and tales of long ago and of the present, of what James did when he was younger and of incidents from her own childhood, she told fairytales and made up stuff when she ran out of things to say. She just kept talking.

All the while she kept her voice gentle but enthusiastic, with highs and lows in just the right places to emphasize this and that. It wasn't just a big tree in the story, it was a biiiiig tree and her voice rose just in the right place and her arm would fly upwards to show how big the tree really was. And James' eyes would open wide and his eyebrows would rise right up almost as big as the tree itself, as he became immersed in her tale, so that it was the most natural thing in the world for him to open his mouth and eat the broth and then eventually, the soup.

As the food went into his starving and malnourished body, the healing began, until by the beginning of the second week, he and his brother were eating full bowls of soup every two hours and still being hungry in between. Fussy eater? Where? Not in our house anymore!

What a transformation! It was simply amazing. My mum fed and fed and fed – and then no more. By the fourth week of Introduction, for the first time ever in his whole life, James was so enthusiastic about his food that he wanted to feed himself!

Now, as we enter week six, he eats on his own and just about anything I put before him. There are definitely things he prefers above others and he doesn't necessarily like everything, but we do manage now to convince him to eat just about anything, with not too much fuss. He devours this beautiful, nutritious, life-giving and life-altering food. I tell everyone now that my boys eat like kings: organic everything and heaps of it.

It beyond amazed me when they wanted to eat the sauerkraut! By week five, they didn't need the juice anymore – they began to just have the kraut with every main meal. They drink that fermented Cod Liver Oil as if it was a spoon of syrup, just on its own, no problem. Same with the EyeQ oil. They devour the Bio-Kult straight off the spoon. They eat veggies, avocado, liver... Before, James gagged when I put an egg anywhere near him. Now I have a hard time stopping him at four a day. Huge bowls of soup, pancakes, veggies, meat, chicken, fermented fish!

And what an adventure when I introduce a new food – oh the excitement, the desire to help prepare it, the dragging of the kitchen chairs over to the sink, the squabbles over who will peel this vegetable or chop up the other, the agony of waiting for it to cook in the oven and oh my gosh, please don't tell them they have to wait for it to cool down when it comes out!

I was just reading this quarter's edition of my *Autism Magazine* and there was an article outlining the research they were doing on fussy eating and how it affected kids on the spectrum and what could be done. I wanted to laugh! I wanted to write to them and tell them to just put an ad for GAPS in their magazine and forget the research and the surveys!

And what effect has all this wonderful nutrition had on James? It has been quite miraculous, and I believe the success has been due to the advice Linda gave us, that we should try to get as much of this food as possible into James – the more he ate the quicker he would heal.

Before we started GAPS, my James had many issues. I wrote them all down before we began the diet and there were 25 that I could think of. They were all typical symptoms that an autistic child would have. We are now entering week six of GAPS and are in stage three of the Introduction Diet and I have crossed *seven* symptoms off my list.

These are: obsession with the washing machine, obsession with electrical cords and power-boards, obsessed with playing at the sinks and with the pump soap, very picky eater, no interest in toys, walks with his chest sticking out and his hands extended up at shoulder level, and uninterested in fine motor work.

We first began to notice a difference at about week three when James started asking to play with play dough – something he was never interested in before. When we gave it to him, he actually played with it and attempted to make things with it, naming them and telling us about them, where before he just held the play dough in his hands and stared ahead, not knowing what to do with it.

Then he started asking to do drawing and painting and cutting with the scissors, whereas before, he would just hold a pen or a pair of scissors and not know what to do.

All the while, as he was doing these new activities, we noticed he had not been near the washing machine, a power cord or the sink in a long while. One day, the washing machine was on and he walked right past it and into the toy room and started playing with the toy drum, like it is supposed to be played with. Usually you couldn't drag him away from the washing machine. It was like a veil had been lifted from his eyes and he all of a sudden discovered, hey, there are toys in this house! It was like he just woke up.

I now often find little towers of blocks around the house that he has built. I might walk into a room and he will be flicking through a book. The other day, he actually rode on his scooter. And oh, the icing on the cake, he has been playing with his brother, Tom. He didn't do any of these things before!

I cried for James before – tears of such sadness for my boy, because darkness was overshadowing his future. Now, barely a day goes by when I still don't cry, but these tears are of such intense gratitude. I am so grateful, firstly and foremost to God, because the knowledge of this diet came to us shortly after heartfelt prayer for help. I am so grateful to Him for placing everything we need to heal, within the bodies of the creatures of this earth and the plants that grow upon it. And I am sorry on behalf of humanity that we have turned away from Him and chosen artificial means with which to nourish ourselves!

I am secondly, so grateful to Dr Natasha, for rediscovering this most valuable diet and being so generous as to share it with the world. I am grateful to Linda Paterson, who has held my hand professionally and been there to answer my myriad of questions. I do believe that our progress would have been slower without her.

I am eternally grateful to my mum – the super Greek grandmother, a natural born-and-gifted feeder and lover of children, from whom I have learned much, and my dad, Papou, who spent endless hours play-ing with my boys, so I could wash ever-growing mounds of dishes and attempt to tidy an increasingly messy house.

Finally, I am ever grateful to my husband John, who passed away seven months before we began GAPS. He resides in my heart now, and I often remind him of the tears of grief he cried for James before he died. I ask him never to forget us before the throne of God and I can feel his prayers for us from heaven mightily.

We sure do have a long way to go and James still has many issues to overcome, which shows that there is still much healing needed. But this is such a ray of hope for us, this wonderful progress in this short time. I now have hope that he may have an opportunity to live as close as possible to a 'normal' life as can be, with friends and meaningful relationships and work.

I would like to encourage all grandparents and friends of parents with autistic children who have embarked upon the GAPS journey. Please help these parents – they will surely need it, for this will probably be one of the most difficult things they will ever do in their lives! Please be there for them in any way you can! And then you will have the most wonderful reward for your generosity – you will have the privilege of personally witnessing the miraculous events which will surely unfold, right before your very eyes. For even though the journey is difficult, it is, undoubtedly, most worthwhile!

A comment from Dr Natasha

What a heart-warming story, thank you Anna! Fussy eating is a very common problem amongst autistic and other GAPS children. It is the first hurdle many parents must overcome before the diet can really be implemented. I used the word 'must' because fussy eating is a major symptom of GAPS. It is not an option to work around this symptom; it has to be dealt with head on. How beautiful it is that the whole family got involved in the work, including the grandparents, God bless them! With such a powerful team involved I am sure that very soon you will have two very healthy sons, a joy to bring up!

4

Ophelia

Key words: childhood anorexia, fussy eating, learning and behavioural problems, vegetarianism

The Pickiest Eater on the Block

There's a cliché about parenting that a lot of people will happily parrot: 'It's so much work!' they'll say in this chipper, reminiscing sort of voice. 'But it's all worth it!' This line of thinking – that parenting can make a person's life more or less 'worth it' and that children are absolute mirrors of their parents' skill at parenting – is something I believed for a very long time. I believed it all the way through my pregnancy, which was a very smug time indeed, because I knew everything! My baby was growing perfectly, fed by my meticulous vegetarian diet consisting of only whole foods. I exercised every day, and walked on back streets to avoid excessive auto exhaust. My baby would be born at home, we would use no drugs or antibiotics or vaccinations, s/he would breastfeed on demand, and co-sleep, and later on would home-school; mine would be the happiest baby in the whole, wide world.

Alex was indeed born at home, a beautiful, normal birth, with no interventions or drugs, and this fit right in with my plan. Only thing was, he arrived three weeks before his due date. At 6 lb 10 oz he seemed just fine, although he was really sleepy. He would barely nurse at all for the first few days, and as I began to explode painfully with milk, the sheer volume would choke him whenever he did latch on.

At about two weeks old, he started waking up five, six or more times per night, and developed horrible 'colic' that would cause him to scream for hours at a stretch. I was so exhausted that I could barely function. Alex was gaining weight okay (and he continued to gain, for his first year of life), but nursing was horribly painful, as were the bizarre shooting pelvic cramps I developed. Post-partum depression was terrible, although I didn't call it that, or even know what it was that made me wake up crying in the night along with my baby. Colic is often due to an 'immature digestive tract,' the books said. But when would it mature?!? ....Parenting was not fitting in with my fantasies.

For six months Alex threw up all the time, and screamed a lot, and slept very little. I knew that lots of babies did this, some worse than ours. But Alex's reflux was just a little bit worse than normal, his screaming just a little louder than many, and now some of his development (sitting, walking, talking) was coming along just a little slower than the other babies we knew. And that's how lots of Alex's challenges continued to evolve – just a little bit more than normal.

Nursing was uncomfortable and painful for years, although I managed to keep at it until just after Alex's third birthday. It seemed necessary, since he barely ate any solid food till he was two. Once he started eating, he craved bread and starch. I'd heard that this was normal, but Alex craved these things more intensely and exclusively than all my friends' babies, especially considering that we never ate refined sugar or flour or junk food. Where did these particular tastes come from??

Weird little behaviours started popping up out of nowhere around when Alex was 22 months: he stopped hugging anyone but me (and even these hugs weren't very cuddly), and he developed antisocial tendencies (crying when people were around; shrinking back from friendly touches; averting his eyes when folks talked; refusing to respond to questions; ignoring people entirely). He got obsessive about things: he hated dust, and he wanted others to repeat activities over and over, and would get more and more agitated when they lost interest in his favourite things (trucks, backhoe loaders, and later storm drains, sewers, puddles, and downspouts... and drawing pictures of all of the above). At around two and a half, he developed an intermittent and sometimes intense aversion to crowds, sometimes even crowds as small as his two parents.

His gastrointestinal state hit a low around his third birthday, when he hadn't gained weight in two years, was having diarrhoea eight times a day, and was waking up at 4a.m. with tummy cramps that made him cry. Removing gluten and dairy from his diet helped somewhat, but it wasn't a cure, and his peculiar eating habits got even more exclusive and peculiar, despite my constant attempts to normalize his food intake and encourage him to try new things. After age three, he never tried anything new.

Over the next three and a half years, Alex's attacks of gastrointestinal distress grew increasingly severe, and sometimes lasted for weeks. These consisted of listlessness and lethargy (he'd lie in bed and stare at the wall, not moving), even further loss of his already small appetite, and unmentionable distress and purging (sometimes vomiting, sometimes diarrhoea, sometimes even while he was asleep).

Each attack was scary, and each time I would research another hazy 'syndrome' about which nobody knows that much, when you get right down to it: Crohn's, Celiac, food intolerance, Irritable Bowel Syndrome. None of the potential diagnoses or their treatments provided helpful ideas. Usually, when I told the paediatrician about the latest attack, she would mention that a stomach bug was 'going around'. Once we got a stool test, but it showed nothing conclusive. After each attack it would take Alex a month to get back to 'normal', which wasn't very good to begin with.

Jeff or I had to be with him at all times, to avoid meltdowns, which were often unavoidable these days anyway. The screaming was intense, long-lasting, and sometimes severe. Between the ages of three and six and a half, he logged countless hours throwing 'fits'. 'Tantrums are normal' everyone, including child psychologists, assured me. But was it really normal for a child to scream over tiny little problems for continuous hours at a stretch?

Alex was growing and developing almost entirely 'normally'... except for all the ways in which he wasn't. The behaviours were growing harder to ignore, and they didn't make sense. There was his non-acceptance of physical affection, varying levels of rigidity and inflexibility (often culminating in the aforementioned hours' worth of explosive screaming fits), near inability to interact with people outside the home, speech delays and bizarre speech patterns and repetitive questioning, having no apparent desire for peer interaction, obsessive toileting habits, inability to play independently, apparent lethargy/depression, tiny stature, bloated belly, compulsive smelling of objects, shirt-chewing, anxiety attacks, pale appearance, very skinny except for a bloated tummy, wanting to be next to a family member at all times, skin rashes...

All these symptoms and many more made it pretty difficult to get through many days. But sometimes there would be marginal improvements – just enough to say, 'Oh, it's just a stage. He'll just grow out of it.' Alex's 'percentile' on the weight/height chart went from high-normal at age one, down to the 10th percentile by age three. Definitely not a big child, but still on the charts. Jeff and I would watch, and try to appreciate his intelligence and artistic creativity, which, while substantial, were often overshadowed by his incredibly challenging 'disposition'. And then he'd regress again, and onward we would stumble.

SOMETHING WAS WRONG! I shoved this intuition away as often as I could, since he was my first kid and I was in denial. How could so much be wrong when I was trying so hard to do everything right?? Everything developed so insidiously, slowly, and non-dramatically. It took me a long time to stop thinking that my life was awful, or that I was a crappy mother, or that Alex was doing all these things to spite me or manipulate me. Things just ramped up until Jeff and I didn't even realize how much our family life was centered around compensating for Alex's explosions and dealing with Alex's behaviours and trying to pretend that everything was okay.

Many people suggested that we get a 'diagnosis' for Alex. But I didn't see exactly how this would help. Maybe Alex would have been called Asperger's, or Pervasive Developmental Disorder Not Otherwise Specified, or as suffering from Social Anxiety or having a paranoid-over-parenting mother. But what's the use of getting him a label if all these most-legitimate-sounding syndromes have no cures, only therapy to help 'manage' the symptoms? In what ways do the labels help a parent address the complexity of the child's mental and physical health? Diagnoses of mental illness sometimes help parents get taken seriously. Maybe, in our case, it might have absolved me of vast amounts of guilt somewhat sooner than later. But currently popular treatments for 'psychiatric' disorders are, at best, notoriously challenging to get 'just right' to positively affect a patient's brain chemistry; and often, at worst, they are completely ineffective or actually make the problems worse. Drugs cause side effects, often very terrible ones. Occupational therapy might make sense for some, to offer basic compensatory strategies to help a person's brain iron out a few quirks. But an effective healing protocol for mental illness? Stories about complete recovery are mighty hard to come by...

I am an unschooler, born and bred. I don't believe in 'normal,' in putting people into little boxes, and labeling them, and trying to make children into another person's idea of what a 'child should be'.

And then I heard about the Specific Carbohydrate Diet. This was in April 2010. We started the diet the next day! At this point, Alex was so anxious that he'd scream if I left the house. He spent a lot of time screaming even when I was *in* the house. He was in the midst of a terrible Attack which was lasting for weeks. He was barely eating anything, he complained about leg cramps, and didn't want to go out.

Prior to the Attack, his diet had already dwindled to the point where Alex would only eat these foods: home-made sourdough gluten-free grain products, eggs, hummus, some fruits, and to a much lesser degree (<1 x week), potatoes, pesto, and sometimes a dairy-free smoothie, and VERY occasionally (<1 x month), broccoli or raw carrots. That's it. He never ate anything else. No vegetables, no soup, no dessert, no broth, no tea, not even chocolate-gluten-free-cake, nothing. Not even if he went for 24 hours without eating would he ever try anything new, unless it was a new kind of bread. The smell, the texture, even the sight of 'new' foods would make him gag. So, beginning a new diet was a daunting prospect. But I didn't see another choice. He was barely eating anything as it was.

To complicate an already disordered eating scenario, I was a lifelong vegetarian, and although I had never forbidden my children meat, we'd never had any in the house – until now.

For the first seven days of the SCD, all Alex would eat was almond bread and eggs. Then he fasted for three days, and had a massive vomiting / diarrhoea / purging extravaganza. After this stressful introduction to the Specific Carbohydrate Diet, Alex was like a changed child – happy, vivacious (!), talkative (!!) and hungry (!!!). My child, who had always had such terrible sensory issues that he couldn't even chew, was eating chunks and textures and tastes. I could barely keep up with his appetite. I started reading the GAPS book, so I made him soups, and tried to come up with other options in between. But on day four of this crazy eating, not knowing better I let him have a little fruit in between his bowls of soup. By the end of the week, he was practically psychotic, at least compared to the happy, hungry little boy I'd had at the table a few days earlier. He wanted more fruit, less soup, and finally no soup at all.

I started freaking out, and after reading more about GAPS, decided to put our whole family on the Introduction Diet. Thing was, Alex was fasting again. He absolutely, positively refused to eat anything but eggs, for about the next seven days. Jeff now started freaking out with me. Alex is a small child. He'd just finished 10 days of near-fasting. He had to eat! We spent the following three weeks in absolute hell, trying to force Alex to eat the three delicious meals that we served him each day. At this point, he stopped wanting even the foods he'd previously liked. It was unbelievably awful!

I spoke with Dr Thomas Cowan, by phone. The basic premise of his advice was: you can't force a child to eat. Eating is all about autonomy. You choose what to feed him, but he chooses what to consume. I thought, great! Yay! That makes so much sense! No more force-feeding, just serve Alex good, wholesome foods, and wait till he's hungry again, and he'll eat them. I mean, I could still remember that time in April when, for four days, I watched him eating like there was no tomorrow... Except that this time, when we stopped with the food coercion, and instead simply served tasty, nutritious meals three times a day, Alex didn't start eating. Not at all, for a week, nothing but the eggs at breakfast. By day seven, the screaming fits were awful. By day eight, it was getting really, really bad. By day nine, he had stopped throwing fits only because, I think, he was too tired to scream.

I cannot explain what it is like to see your child actually weaken in hunger, and yet refuse to eat the foods that you are offering with love and intention to make him well. I remember feeling this kind of despair when Alex was newborn and wouldn't nurse for the first two weeks. Then and now, I was terrified: why wouldn't he eat?! This is what dying people do!

Finally, on Day 12 of the current fast, Dr Cowan informed me that Alex had broken the record for anorexic eating among his entire paediatric clientele. This was not a trend that I wanted to continue, so my resolve broke down. I basically began serving Alex eggs for every single meal. I tried to blend up meats and veggies and fats and put them in too, but essentially what Alex ate for the next several months was eggs. He revived a bit on this egg diet, definitely. But he wasn't doing spectacularly. And by the time the end of August rolled around, he was starting to refuse even his 'egg things'.

Hearing so many good things about coconut kefir, I started giving this to him, about ? cup the first time. Strangely, although he would refuse delicious food at every meal, he would - very grudgingly - take supplements like kefir and green juice. He went ballistic for a week on coconut kefir and threw so many tantrums that I stopped it for a few days. And all the time his appetite seemed to be slipping away. There was not enough food going in. I felt pretty strongly that non-food supplements would be a complicated, expensive rabbit hole that rarely cure children fully of anxiety / autism / etc. (especially in the absence of enough nourishing food). And it didn't make sense to stop the kefir, because it's got all these probiotics. Any reaction should be a healing one, since it's definitely not some terrible, indigestible food.

Alex stopped pooping, so we started doing enemas every day... This is when I truly began to examine my child's eating habits. Will take supplements. Won't eat meat, any at all, nor cooked veggies. Will eat fermented veggies (proving that chewing isn't entirely the issue). Cuts food into tiny, infinitesimal pieces ($1/2$ of an avocado into 72 pieces, for example). Picks out 'chunks' and arranges them decoratively on his plate. Eats incredibly small bites. Almost seems to reduce his portion size progressively, at every meal. Tells me he's full when he hasn't eaten all day. Craves sweets, nut breads, anything that looks like food he used to eat. Isn't growing, hardly at all. Goes at his preferred food with an obsession that just doesn't make sense, given how often he spurns super-delicious meals (even when he's hungry) which his brother gobbles down with relish... I looked up ANOREXIA in the dictionary. ... and then I slammed the figurative dictionary closed. My son needed to get over this eating disorder - preferably tomorrow, but definitely soon!

I researched deficiencies caused by long-term vegetarian diets. Zinc seemed like a good thing to try in the short term, if only for the placebo effect. And eggs, the one obsessive food that Alex was hanging onto for dear life, had to go. I'm writing flippantly about this in retrospect. At the time, I was so, so incredibly worried and stressed and unsure that removing eggs - his One Nourishing Food - was the right choice!

What next? Well, for 10 days, Alex ate: fermented veggies, green juice, and ? teaspoonfuls of coconut kefir. Oh, and his zinc. That is it! He absolutely refused the meals I set before us. Once again, he got weaker and weaker. Once again, after the first week, he stopped screaming, and just sort of sat around listlessly. By the tenth day, he was so hungry, and so hurting, and so little, that I just wanted so badly to feed him waffles, and pancakes, and fruit, and everything his body was craving - the way heroin addicts long for their fix...

On that tenth night, he couldn't fall asleep. His mind was racing, he said, and he was so anxious that he just wanted to lie on top of me. I offered, for the hundredth time, a bowl of soup. And the miracle was that on this night he said: "I'll try it!" My husband and I sat there, spoon-feeding him, and crying. He gagged some, and had trouble chewing, but he ate the first bowl. Then he wanted another. Then he said he was full, but that he wished he wasn't because it tasted so good! And then he fell asleep.

We were not yet out of the woods. For five days, Alex continued to gag and mostly refuse food and sit, in a withered state, on the couch. He was losing weight, and not eating enough, and sometimes accepting soup and other times saying he would not eat unless it was the same soup we had yesterday, and not eating meat, and... and... and. It was more of the same obsessions, just with some soup going in every so often.

I imagine that every child is different, some more and many less extremely picky than ours. But in our case, my husband and I felt like we had to get more nourishing food in, and we couldn't rely on Alex's hunger mechanisms that were, for all intents and purposes, broken. All that we could think of was to appeal to what cognition Alex could muster, and use our status as amateur psychologists. Starting that day, coaching Alex became a full-time task. One of us had to take Alex 's younger brother, and the other one of us had to sit at the table, solidly, patiently, for hours. Jeff was incredibly, amazingly, persistent and kind. The script went kind of like this. "Alex, it's so hard right now. Your brain is playing tricks on you, and those Bad microbes are telling your body not to eat these foods. But we know that these foods will heal you. These are the foods that will help you. They don't taste good to you now, but that's okay. It's okay to eat them even though they don't taste good, because sometime soon they will. For now, you need to make yourself eat them. It might make you gag, and your brain will tell you to eat tiny pieces, but you can do it. You can take normal bites. We're here to help you. That's our job." And on, and on, and on, and on. I was beat, from trying to do this during the week with Alex and his younger brother. So Jeff mostly sat with him that first weekend, for hours. It was probably four days, but it felt like two years, at least.

Then he finally ate a hamburger for the first time! It felt like we had reached a new point of progress. He was eating meat!! Soon after, Alex began eating 2 lb of meat per day, all dipped in extra fat. He gained 5 ? lb in 13 days! We didn't bring eggs back into his diet for another several weeks. When he'd been eating solidly, for 10 days or so, he finally was able to poop by himself (I'd done 60 consecutive days of enemas, by this time). There was lots of diarrhoea, and also lots of normal poops, and also lots of weird ones.

Here we were in October, six months after starting the diet – and this was the real beginning of GAPS. True, we'd strictly avoided all 'illegal' foods before. But now the nourishment was finally going in, as many different foods as we could, no matter what it took.

It's so hard to know with our kids what is 'best'. Most of the time, we can never know. But it was increasingly clear to Jeff and me that once Alex 's hunger kicked in (the real hunger, not cravings for eggs or starch), he also had to keep eating, and *on our terms*. This may sound cruel, but it also felt like a matter of life and death. A six-year-old who has just been fasting for 10 days needs to NOT DO that anymore – and not only that, we had to prevent another slide backwards into his bizarrely easy default of MOSTLY NOT EATING.

It became clear (although the lines are always fuzzy) that often, when Alex says that he's 'full', he really means he's in discomfort, or that something's actually hurting, or that he Just Doesn't Want To Eat, with all of his messed-up-microbes, with every GAPS fibre of his little being. I have this theory that when adults are starting GAPS, and they feel really horrible, with die-off, etc., they analyze their health to the maximum. They discover that various foods feel better or worse than others, or they realize how their fat absorption is compromised, and they figure out ways to get nourishment from the few foods that currently work for them, while trying to heal the gut and be able to comfortably tolerate more variety. I wonder if, for our kids, they have all this discomfort too, but mostly no way to articulate what they're feeling. With Alex, I'm sure he was reacting to foods, and all that fat, and maybe everything that we were pushing him to eat. But in our case, I had no way to know, and no time to be choosy. We needed to trust that he could push through maybe dozens of these initial unpleasant reactions, and push through, in order to get to a point where we were stable. Perhaps this is more messy than the reasoned-adult-patient approach, but I'm hopeful that it has the same result, eventually: healing the gut.

So. Once Alex had started eating lots of meat (our particular personal challenge), we coasted for a few days – but I also realized, we had to keep pushing. This had been the third time Alex had fasted, and I didn't want to make the mistakes I'd made last time. I tried to imagine: what do we want our meals to consist of? And then I tried to make our meals look like that. I know that at some point, we'll be able to follow all of our intuitions and just eat when we're hungry; but for now, Jeff and I had to come up with A Plan. Once all the 'required' items were consumed at a meal, Alex could have seconds or thirds of whatever part of the meal he was enjoying most (meat or veggies).

Here was our basic menu:

Breakfast: Some kind of meat, some kind of veggie, lots of fat, cup of broth, a fermented vegetable, young coconut kefir (YCK).

Lunch: Fermented vegetable, large bowl of soup with veggies and broth, sometimes meat and sometimes not, YCK.

Snack: Green juice (celery, cucumber, lettuce, and sometimes cabbage).

Dinner: Some kind of meat, some kind of veggie, lots of fat, a fermented vegetable, YCK, sometimes more broth.

Toward a More Comprehensive Theory of GAPS Picky Eaters

(Or, what I wished I known the first time Alex practiced self-starvation, back in April)

1. These kids can go for a LONG time without eating. Obviously, we'd rather they eat, but I'm starting to think that this *fasting has therapeutic benefits* that we can't quite fathom yet. If I had it to do over, I wouldn't have given myself the additional stress (on top of all that I already had!) of panicking when Alex went for weeks without eating. I think we need to trust that eventually they will eat, when the cleansing, or whatever it is, has run its course.

2. Once they start eating, we're often so relieved and shaky from what just happened, that we can be tempted to let them eat whatever they want. But GAPS kids are not fit to make their own choices. *We* have to choose for them the foods that will heal them.

3. Progress won't be linear. The first night when they start eating, maybe they'll eat the soup – the next day, they might refuse it, and want chicken, and we'll rush to make it for them. I think it's so, so incredibly important that we don't let them dictate their own food choices! These choices come from their sensory issues and obsessions; they are GAPS symptoms, and the only way we're going to heal these things is by making sure that the pillars of our diet go in (veggies, fats, meats, broths, ferments). We have to be compassionate, and parental, but change the dynamics of the power in the family: from now on *we decide what to serve*, and tell them how important it is that they make themselves eat it.

4. I think one of the most important things we can do, once the child starts eating, is to stand firm in the foods we serve, and constantly mix it up. Different meats. Different veggies. Different cooking techniques. Different ferments. Nothing the same, from one day to the next. It is important because, as their bodies adapt to the new foods, *they try to latch onto new obsessive items*. Breaking the obsessive patterns probably takes a different amount of time for every child, but I know that at the two-month-mark we are far from healed; in Alex's case the obsessions were so bad that we spent years feeding him eggs on gluten-free toast for breakfast

every single day, because if we missed a day there was hell to pay…
We have to give ourselves and our kids time and compassion with
this whole process!

5. *We need to up the ferments gradually*, because these will keep
   fighting the battle with the bad microbes in our kids' guts.

6. *Expect that the child will regress.* Decide how to deal with this
   when it happens, not if. Alex has had many episodes, since he
   started eating, where we've had to sit with him, and talk him
   through taking a bite of food. We tell him, we know your tastes
   haven't changed right now for this particular food, but it's okay.
   Remember the hamburger? The tastes will change. These foods
   will heal you. These foods need to go in. It's one of the most
   important things you can possibly do. We will never force you to
   eat, ever again, but you need to force yourself… These episodes are
   draining and awful and confusing and sad, and they keep happening. But I'm sure he will get over them, in time. For now, we have
   to budget many hours per week to counseling him through.

7. *Try to keep in sight the way that you eventually want mealtimes
   to be.* Eventually it won't be this crazy. Eventually our kids will
   eat. Eventually, there will be joy in food, and the lack of it right
   now is not because of the food, anyway – it's because of this darn
   leaky gut…

8. *We are incredible parents*! We don't hear it very often, because
   our kids can't say it, and most of the rest of the world thinks we're
   'nuts' (plus, they notice our often-obnoxious children). But we
   have to know this, and keep telling each other, because otherwise,
   hardly anyone will. I so appreciated all the encouragement folks
   sent (and are sending!) my way, and it's helping me through the
   rough spots. And the most important thing is that I believe in
   myself and my family and my kid.

9. Know that we'll never know enough to be sure about all this. We
   have to hone our intuition and our intellect and then plunge in.
   We'll be learning every second, as we go along.

Here are some things I think are true:

– GAPS is a healing diet, requiring the consumption of what I think of
  as the pillars of our diet: meats, broths, non-sweet cooked veggies,

fats, fermented vegetables and pure green juice, with no sweet ingredients; optionally, eggs and fermented dairy.
- Optional on GAPS: sweet veggies, raw veggies, nuts, fruits, honey.
- Many GAPS kids, once started on the diet, almost miraculously find that their tastes change, allowing them to enjoy almost every new food that's put in front of them (with minimal, normal-style taste preferences).
- Many other GAPS kids are extremely picky to start; and once on the diet, they either fast at the beginning, refuse to eat until some favoured food is served, or latch onto new favourite foods with the same obsessive fervour they had for their former, now-illegal foods.

We GAPS parents are already dealing with huge to massive behaviour/health challenges with our kids, and it might seem easy to discount picky eating as something that isn't pertinent to the whole GAPS pathology. But I think that the picky eating is a huge symptom, which presents because of the GAPS brain's toxicity, much like other autistic, depressive, ADHD, etc. symptoms. Of course, we all know that we can't heal our kids with a healing diet if the kids won't eat. So the question becomes, if we have one of these picky to super-picky eaters, how do we get the food in??

Options:
- ABA techniques
- Force feeding
- Letting them eat whatever legal foods they want, whenever they want, on the theory that At Least They're Eating.
- Serving them the good foods their bodies need, knowing that while we can't know exactly what they need, it's pretty darn close. And if they don't eat these foods, tough – this is what's for dinner...

1. ABA does not work for many kids. If it did for yours, great, read no further. It did not work, no way no how, for my son. If you tried to get one spoonful of broth into him in exchange for a bite of another food, well, then he could and would scream for two hours straight in protest – and not ever eat the broth.

2. Force-feeding might work for some kids, but it sure didn't work for mine. Encouragement, threats, rewards, punishments: these complicated our lives for three solid weeks of trying and I wanted to die. Plus, my son wasn't eating measurably more – one day he sat at the table for eight hours rather than eat breakfast!

3. Letting kids eat whatever legal foods they want – usually a few foods that resemble their previous diet, like eggs, almond bread, certain meats, smoothies – might work for some people. But usually there is at least one food group missing: ferments, maybe veggies, or lots of fats. And nuts are a pretty advanced food for a weakened digestive system, and seem like they could really slow down the healing process, especially if there's yeast in our kids' bodies. Many kids can probably continue on this limited diet pretty indefinitely. We went for six months. But my son is small, and he wasn't gaining weight. He wasn't making huge cognitive gains, although there were small ones. He was marginally less anxious, but extremely difficult to live with. Was he getting better? All in all, he wasn't progressing very far or fast. Could he have healed this way? Maybe, but I didn't want to wait until he was 25 to find out. More and more, I think that we have to overcome this picky eating, as a fundamental GAPS symptom, before our kids can heal.

4. So now we come to the final option, which I now believe might be our only chance at healing our kids relatively quickly. Their little systems are resilient, but we need to get the foods in there. All of the foods. The meats are important. The broths are healing. The fats are essential, especially for their little toxic brains. The cooked vegetables help balance out all these flesh-based healing foods. I'm pretty convinced we need the ferments to go in, at most every meal, for the rest of our lives (this is the only sustainable, affordable, and complete way of introducing enough probiotics for our kids to both fight the bad bugs and heal up their insides, and then actually feel well). The green juice, depending upon the child, might be nearly a requirement, for detoxifying all the crazy stuff that the die-off will stir up.

ALL THE OTHER GAPS FOODS – fermented dairy, fruit, nuts, sweet veggies, etc.– are non-essentials. Our kids could go for years eating just ferments, meat, fats, broths, cooked veggies, and green juice. These are incredibly nutritious, and can heal them, and maybe in a couple of years, we can add the other stuff in.

What is going on with our kids and their near-anorexic tendencies? You might say that your picky child isn't as bad as mine. But what happens when you take away their obsession foods, the ones they 'like'? What happens if you serve your kids chunks, instead of a smoothie? What happens if you give them chicken instead of pork? If they're anything like my son, they will refuse to eat it. And they can hold out. And hold out. Definitely, they can wait to eat until the next meal, they can often wait for 24 hours, and – I know from experience – sometimes they can go for at least 12 days!

I have a theory that we've got two issues to deal with: GAPS toxicity symptoms (pickiness, sensory stuff like gagging, wanting smooth/crispy foods, food refusal/obsession behaviours), and then the habits that form around these symptoms. You've got a kid who before GAPS ate peanut butter and jelly on white bread, with the bread cut into hexagons, plus ice cream and potato chips and scrambled eggs. You put this kid on GAPS, and even if the sensory issues are subsiding, you'd never know it, because he's not healed enough to let go of his obsessions, and he's already latched onto GAPS-legal almond bread (or carrots, or whatever), plus scrambled eggs and smoothies... .and this is now all he'll eat. GAPS-legal, but definitely not a nourishing-enough diet. Certainly not enough to support their bodies in dealing with heightened die-off if we introduce healing foods like kefir, cod liver oil, raw fermented dairy, etc. We have to shift both the foods that our kids are eating and the behaviours that accompany them...

Helping my child learn how to eat, in order to institute the protocol that will heal everything else, has been the hardest thing I have ever begun – and our journey is far from over. The most amazing, wild, and awesome sight is my formerly-food-addicted, super-super-picky eater learning to like food. And by this I mean, FOOD, in all its varied forms, not just the two or three 'acceptable' items to which he used to cling for dear life and not really enjoy at all. For so long, I felt so bad about the idea of 'taking away' his 'favourite foods.' I thought: how could I make my child's diet even more restricted?? And now... I feel like such a great mother (definitely with flaws, but great nonetheless), simply because Jeff and I have given Alex this gift, to learn to eat a less restricted diet than he's ever eaten in his life. The restrictions used to be imposed by himself, and his toxic brain. Now, he's eating foods that are healing him, and enjoying such a wide range of foods that it almost breaks my heart. On the good days we keep a close eye on him, to sort of make sure it's not a Cinderella at Midnight.

Meanwhile, Alex got amnesia. "What did I eat, before I first started eating meat?" Alex asked me recently, a few weeks after he Started Eating. 'Well, not much!' I told him. "Remember? You used to eat eggs, and 'egg things,' pretty much." "Nothing else?" Alex asked, amazed, like he was remembering something that happened years and years ago, only just vaguely. "Did I eat any vegetables?" I remembered back, over all those years' and years' worth of refused meals – and quickly quenched that thought. "Hardly any", I said. "Remember? You'd started eating sauerkraut, but no other vegetables, really." "Why?" Alex asked, wonderingly. "Why didn't I? If I was hungry, could I? If I'd wanted to, couldn't I eat meat and vegetables? Could I eat soup?"

I looked at his little face, so confused by these strange memories, and I took advantage of the way he lets me kiss him now, most of the time, right on the top of his fuzzy blond head...

Yes, my kiddo! Let this fade. I can't tell you how thrilled I am, every day that we get farther away from all the thousands of times I've watched my baby, sitting in his chair, refusing food. As you keep eating, I am so much less fearful of the painful symptoms that still wrack your body. This time, I know that you can kick these microbes out on their asses, because you are eating! Goddamn it, you are EATING! These foods will nourish you, and make you well, and some-day you won't remember these early years at all. You won't remember your anxiety, because it won't possess you anymore. You won't need to chew your shirt and smell everything and hide your face from people, because your brain won't make you do it anymore. You won't have horrible and crippling stomach pains. You won't remember all the ways we've had to learn and grow and work like crazy in order to heal a six-and-a-half-year-old anorexic.

AND FOR THIS, I AM UTTERLY AND WEEPILY THANKFUL!

You can read more on Ophelia's website www.lifeisapalindrome.com

A comment from Dr Natasha

What a heart-warming story! Every parent with a fussy eater should read it. What Ophelia and her husband have accomplished with their son Alex is no less than 'climbing up Everest and then climbing down it on the other side'. The experience and insight they gained is precious and will help many families to heal their children. Thank you, Ophelia, for sharing your story! You and your husband are wonderful parents, and one day your son himself will tell you that!

5

Brenda Scott

real-food farmer in Molalla, Oregon

Key words: autoimmunity, malabsorption and poor growth, digestive problems, sugar addiction, gum disease, heart palpitations, thyroid problems, neurological symptoms

The six of us have been on this diet for one year now. It all started with going gluten-free for a year. We had attempted gluten-free twice before that, but never whole-heartedly. One night our son Isaac, (seven at the time) cried at the dinner table and asked why he didn't grow, even though he ate so much. And why the other kids on his soccer team were so much taller than him ... This prompted our whole-hearted effort towards gluten-free eating.

Isaac was born at 26 weeks gestation, and since he started at only 1 lb 12 oz, he's always been 'catching up.' We had multiple tests done on him for lots of different things, and we never got any answers. He had a tube in his nose (an NG Tube) for several months, and he had a G-Tube in his belly for a few years. He still didn't grow well. The two years before we went gluten-free, he stayed at 39 lb – for two years straight ... The year we went gluten-free, he went up to 41 lb. Not much, but a significant jump considering the lack of growth the year before. He had acid reflux and a low appetite. Many times we would have a hard time getting him to eat much at all. He didn't appreciate 'real' food and would not eat eggs.

Our second born, Kaleb, was a sugar addict. We'd often find him in the pantry stealing chocolate chips, or we'd find a bunch of Hershey Kiss wrappers hiding behind the canned foods. He would fuss about not getting dessert. He was a moody, up-and-down kid.

Our third son, Noah, has been lactose intolerant since we adopted him when he was 14 months old. He has also been little for his age (short plus underweight). He has also struggled with moodiness more severely than any of the other kids. He also had severe constipation and would often cry when he had to go to the bathroom, and would 'hold it' so that he didn't have to deal with the pain.

Ruby, our adopted daughter, has only ever been able to tolerate raw milk; pasteurised milk products and all infant formulas made her vomit. She was a sugar addict, especially when it came to chocolate. She's a big eater and big for her age (she's three and wears the same size clothes as Noah, who is seven). She didn't really NEED a new diet, but we thought it wouldn't hurt her.

My husband was pretty healthy except that he had some weight to lose, had back issues every now and then, often had low energy and suffered from psoriasis.

Then there was my health. Our bodies are so complex, and my body was reminding me daily how complex it really is! Here were my issues:

- Often weak, even as a little kid. Tested for hypoglycaemia and showed up 'borderline' multiple times.
- Often felt blood sugar 'lows' in between breakfast and lunch and in between lunch and dinner. I had a secret stash of chocolate in the pantry to get me through those lows.
- Anaemic.
- Felt like a 'rag doll' many times – like it just took too much strength to lift up my own body.
- Acid reflux just about every night.
- Chest pains, heart palpitations and periodic numbness in my left arm; once my arm was numb for 11 hours, when I spent some time in the hospital ER with no answers found.
- Tummy aches often.
- Diarrhoea often.
- Constipation often.
- Numbness in my chin and jaw for a couple of months.
- Strange muscle issues. Sometimes when I would grip something, the grip wouldn't stop – my hand stayed stuck in that position.
- Very painful muscle cramps in my legs at night.

- Random itchiness. All over.
- Arthritis in my hands and feet.
- Weak immune system. I caught everything that was going around.
- High serotonin. My dad has *Carcinoid Syndrome*, a familial cancer that involves tiny tumours that produce lots of serotonin. I was sensitive to all of the high-serotonin foods, especially tomatoes, berries, peppers, and avocados.
- Canker sores. Or whatever you call them. Little tiny bumps all over inside my mouth, often.
- The 'butterfly rash' at times (Lupus?) and 'flushing' in my face whenever I'd eat something spicy or I'd get stressed out.
- Ear aches. It felt like food was going up inside my right ear and it hurt.
- High ANA (auto nuclear antibodies), which meant I had some kind of autoimmune disease.
- High thyroid antibodies but normal thyroid hormone levels. So my own body was attacking my thyroid. My dad also has thyroid cancer and has had surgery plus radiation.
- Gum disease. I brushed my teeth well, at least twice a day, but I still had receding and very red gums.
- Had some weight to lose.

Gluten-free helped, but it wasn't enough... My arthritis and acid reflux went away, but I still felt weak and shaky. Isaac gained a little weight, but not enough. I was still catching everyone's colds and sore throats. I started looking into what our next options were, since gluten-free obviously wasn't enough for us....I was curious about my high serotonin (Isaac had high serotonin also), and when I googled 'kids and high serotonin', everything I read was about kids with autism – so I started searching for the perfect autism diet, thinking we had something in common with autistic kids. I first read *Breaking the Vicious Cycle* about the SCD diet. When I began googling SCD, I found out about GAPS. It was just what we needed. It was what I believed was 'healthy eating' anyways... .So began our journey...

After a year on the GAPS Diet, I am happy to report:
Isaac is now 46 lb and growing. He has so much more energy and his

face has more colour. His acid reflux is gone. His appetite is WAY up! He can easily eat five eggs for breakfast!

Kaleb is no longer a sugar addict and his moodiness has subsided. He has become an eight-year-old 'teacher' about real food to everyone he knows!

Noah is up to 40 lb and growing. He does not struggle with constipation any more at all! We're still working on his moodiness.

Ruby continues to grow but is no longer addicted to chocolate.

A ll of our kids started eating their vegetables better not long after being on this diet. Taking out the sugar really helped their taste buds to start appreciating good food!

My husband has lost about 40 lb, hasn't had back issues at all anymore, has more energy than he remembers 'ever' having, and feels GREAT.

And me...Every single symptom on that list is GONE when I stick to the GAPS diet. There have been a couple of times that we have 'cheated' and my symptoms came back with a vengeance. But when we stick to GAPS, I am able to live symptom-free, full of energy, and I feel healthy!!! I have not had my blood tests redrawn lately (ANA, thyroid and serotonin), but I wouldn't be surprised if they are lower as well, since all of the symptoms they caused me are GONE! I can now eat tomatoes and peppers with no problem. I haven't tried avocados again because of the severity of my previous reaction, but someday I'd love to try them again...I have lost about 40 lb – from a size 10 or 12 to a 2. I am small-framed, so I finally feel like ME!

I love this diet! My family loves this diet and I think SO many people can be healed by it! I believe in this diet, because I've seen it work for my family!

You can read more on Brenda's blog www.wellfedhomestead.com

A comment from Dr Natasha

It is wonderful to see how so many seemingly unrelated health problems can disappear due to a simple change in diet! This family of six all had different health challenges: from autoimmunity to hormonal and neurological symptoms. But what united them all were digestive problems. And as the digestive system started to heal in every family member, other symptoms and problems started melting away as well. All diseases do truly begin in the gut! Thank you, Brenda, for sharing your family's story with the world!

6

Nichole Sawatzky

Key words: FPIES (Food Protein Induced Enterocolitis Syndrome), multiple food allergies, eczema, non-convulsive seizures

It is with great pleasure that I share Ellie's story. I can only pray that it helps provide hope and encouragement for other moms dealing with similar struggles.

Ellie was 'colicky' from birth. Exclusively breastfed, she was filling her diapers with blood by 10 weeks old. She was diagnosed with Milk/Soy Protein Intolerance (milk and soy allergy) and placed on an amino acid (elemental) formula. At about eight months of age we began solid foods in an effort to 'weigh things down', and she began bizarre symptoms to every food introduced. Her reactions to everything from rice cereal to bananas included profuse vomiting, severe diarrhoea, manic moods, fever, lethargy and an acidic diaper rash that never went away. She underwent a lengthy amount of tests and procedures, and by 10 months old her diagnosis changed to Food Protein Induced Enterocolitis Syndrome – FPIES (allergy to food).

We were told that she would likely 'outgrow' her condition by age one, or perhaps two. She remained on the elemental formula, and her symptoms worsened. Vomiting was random and often, her stool was extremely constipated, and chronic upper respiratory symptoms kept her wheezing. She developed food aversion, a distended belly, and full-body eczema. She was scoped, biopsied, x-rayed, and given a colonoscopy. Traditional allergy testing (blood and skin prick) showed nothing. Her diagnosis was expanded to include colitis, and sugar intolerance (disaccharidase deficiency). Her skin became so sensitive that she did not tolerate diaper creams, diapers, crayons, bath soap, or stickers on her skin. All induced vomiting, diarrhoea, and shock-like symptoms that were frightening. On occasion she also had hives and swollen eyes.

At 16 months old the allergist conducted patch testing (skin sensitivity testing) which resulted in a scar on her back where corn had been tested. We were told to immediately wean her from the elemental formula which had a corn base, and to feed her home-made almond milk because there is no formula in existence without corn. Our instructions were to move quickly getting other foods into her diet, but to allow for one month of nutrient deficiency before being concerned.

I knew that she would not just suddenly be able to eat food. Not knowing what else to do, we stopped the formula and began giving her almond milk as instructed. And she stopped eating. Every third bottle she vomited uncontrollably and she battled dehydration. She lost 22 ounces almost immediately; I began watching her starve. My mommy-heart ached, and this was the turning point. I suddenly remembered a doctor and a book that was loaned to me when she was born, and I searched the internet. Multiple intolerances, leaky gut, lack of bile, Ileal Lymphoid Nodular Hyperplasia, Non-Specific Colitis and it was all falling into place. All FPIES, and also all GAPS. Ellie needed food NOW, but the fear was crippling. I had been warned to stay away from high protein foods because she would most certainly react, and the GAPS Introduction Diet started with meat broth. So, not knowing what else to do, I sent an email to Dr Campbell-McBride in hopes of finding help where there was none.

What I received from Dr Campbell-McBride was hope, and with that we began Ellie on the introduction diet. It took us approximately four tough weeks to wean Ellie from her formula and start stage one of GAPS. Within 24 hours of her last formula bottle she went from an autism evaluation referral to saying six new words. Within three months she had caught up on all milestones and regained all weight lost. Her non-convulsive seizures stopped entirely.

For 16 months we struggled to help Ellie heal. She was unable to progress past stage one, with zucchini being her only tolerated vegetable. Finally after continual removal of environmental toxins, the help of a GAPS Practitioner, and most importantly lots of time, she is moving forward. She is now three and has a handful of vegetables she can tolerate. She has not had any FPIES type reaction in over a year, and is thriving beyond belief. She is joyful, energetic, and a contemplative chatterbox. She dances, twirls, and sings all day long. And she eats real food. No cough, no sunken eyes, no unexplained vomiting, and no milestone delays. Instead, she wakes up laughing.

We don't know how long it will take Ellie to find complete healing, or move through the stages of GAPS, but that is ok; because now she eats real food, and now she has hope.

Thank you will never say enough!

A comment from Dr Natasha

FPIES (Food Protein Induced Enterocolitis Syndrome) is a fairly new diagnosis, but the number of patients is growing and they are typically infants in their first two years of life. These children test 'allergic' to almost all protein on the planet. They vomit food that is given to them, have diarrhoea and often fail to thrive. The key to treatment is not to avoid all protein (and give the child synthetic substitutes), but to focus on healing and sealing the gut lining with the GAPS Introduction Diet. Once the gut starts healing, food allergies start disappearing one after another, and the child starts thriving. Ellie has a bright future now; she is already a delight to her family and will continue recovering until she is completely healthy. What a wonderful story, thank you Nichole! You can follow this story on a blog: Elliebellyupdates.com.

7

K.H.

Key words: food allergies, failure to thrive, ME (Myalgic Encephalomyelitis), CFS (Chronic Fatigue Syndrome), poor immunity, candida

When my son was born he was quite small but he was on the 10th percentile. I was breastfeeding him exclusively for a year. This was because every time I tried to introduce new foods he would have a reaction e.g. runny nose, being spaced out and the food would come out undigested in his stools (i.e. raw carrots). I have ME/CFS, so I have many health issues including food sensitivities. After my experience with my daughter who is three years older, I was aware that he would probably have inherited all my food sensitivities and more.

I followed the weaning guidelines from LaLeche League for children who are prone to allergies. This involved waiting as long as possible to wean and then once the child has teeth, they can be weaned onto solid foods, which they can hold in their hands and feed themselves. This meant I was giving him raw carrot sticks and cucumber sticks to start with. I now realize that these are very hard to digest and that was why he could not tolerate them. On the positive side I think it was good for him to delay weaning as long as possible, as his digestion was so sensitive. La Leche League was the only place where I could find support for long-term breastfeeding and which had accessible information about allergy prevention.

When he was one, I got him weighed at his yearly check-up with the health visitor; she found that he was very underweight for his age and not even on the chart. The health visitor was very concerned and we had to have monthly weight checks where I was advised to feed him lots of bread, cereal and milk. I tried all these things but he reacted to them all by being very spaced out and having thick green snot coming from his nose. When we stopped these items and he was back on the breast milk, he was symptom-free. The breastfeeding counsellor at LaLeche League was very supportive as well and kept listening to me and helping me to find my own solutions and not judging me, which I felt the health visitor was doing.

I felt deeply worried but didn't know what to do. As a family we had been on an anti-candida diet for 10 years and were used to excluding wheat, dairy, sugar and yeast from our diet. This prevented us from getting very ill, but as soon as we came off it the underlying issues came back. By chance, a friend recommended the book by Dr Natasha Campbell-McBride on the GAPS Diet. I had read this book and found it really inspiring, but could not figure out how to do the diet, as it was so different from our mainly vegetarian anti-candida diet. Fortunately I had a telephone consultation with Dr Natasha and her report really helped me to understand how to do the diet.

I made some chicken stock and cooked some carrots and courgettes in it. I then fed this to my son and he ate them and was symptom-free. In fact, he thrived on this diet! Although we did not follow Dr Natasha's guidelines exactly, he did make good progress and slowly, slowly put on weight. After being on the GAPS Diet for three years he is hardly ever ill and weight-wise is on the 10th percentile.

This was in sharp contrast to my daughter who was always having colds and chest infections. I was always worried that she would have to take antibiotics, and then I would have even more health issues to worry about. She was also constantly craving processed carbohydrates, such as gluten-free bread and pasta. So, after my son and I have been on the GAPS Diet for a year, we decided to put her on the GAPS Diet as well. She did get worse at first, but after a few months she was much better. Now she is hardly ever ill, and when she does get a cold or tummy infection it's gone within 24 hours. Before the GAPS Diet often we could not go out, as the slightest little chill meant that she would catch a cold that lasted for months.

My health is much better, I have lots of energy and many symptoms that I have had for years have improved. The symptoms that have improved include less brain fog, not having pains in my face when it gets cold, putting on weight and a much stronger immune system, very few colds and sore throats. The GAPS Diet has changed our lives and made sure that we are now healthy most of the time!

I am aware though, that we can't move off the GAPS Diet at all, because when we try to do it all our symptoms come back. At the recent Weston A. Price Conference in London I discovered that we haven't completed all the steps properly, such as doing the Introductory phase of the diet and taking the juices. We did the introductory SCD diet, which is quite different and did not suit us so much, as it included lots of fruit jelly. It was only at this conference that I realized that there was a GAPS website gaps.me and yahoo groups. So, doing the GAPS Introduction diet taking the juices is our next step.

We are not completely healed yet, but the huge improvements in our health have been very life-changing and boosting. Thank you for all your help!

A comment from Dr Natasha

Thank you, K.H., for your story! Weaning a baby is a very important step; babies with abnormal gut flora can react quite badly if inappropriate solids are introduced – their mental and physical development can be seriously affected. So K.H. was quite right to be careful and not rush into it. Her own health problems made her aware of what food can do to our health.

And her daughter – there are many children like that, who are not very ill but are not healthy either. They need help as well, and usually all that is required to restore their immune system is proper home-made food.

8

Nancy

Key words: Chronic Fatigue Syndrome, malabsorption, lack of growth and low weight, digestive problems, food allergies, moody and temperamental behaviour, lack of stamina, underachieving at school, headaches, depression

I have had Chronic Fatigue Syndrome since 1992, and in the early years it was very, very disabling. Over the years I have tried numerous alternative therapies and have had some success with improving my symptoms. When I was married the doctors assured me that it was safe to have children and that my condition was unlikely to affect our children.

Before conceiving, I started with *Nourishing Traditions*, eating a healthy traditional diet. Our first daughter was born in 2000 and our second in 2001, and the first year and a half of their lives they were healthy. But then they fell into what I now know is the classic pattern of a GAPS child. After weaning, they both reacted to cow milk. They developed nasal congestion with thick mucus severe enough to make it hard for them to breathe at night. They had trouble sleeping and developed painful sores under their noses from all of the mucous. We switched them to raw goat's milk which worked for a few years, and then they started to react to that, so they went dairy-free.

Then, over time, their symptoms got worse and more diverse. Our younger daughter started having migraine-like headaches almost every day. Her stomach hurt, she had unusual fatigue, and she was moody and temperamental. She spent hours on the couch feeling miserable. We often came home early from birthday parties, the swimming pool, festivals and other kid events because she didn't feel well. In my searching to improve my own health I had discovered that I was gluten intolerant, so I put her on a gluten-free diet, and that seemed to help. She was better, but not well. So, I kept searching for other food allergens. But nothing seemed to make her truly well. Her symptoms came and went in a way that made it hard to figure out what was making her so sick. Every little speck of cross contamination of either gluten or dairy caused a big flare of symptoms. We couldn't eat out without her getting sick. She was falling behind in school and was having immense trouble learning to read.

Her sister seemed to be doing fine on just a dairy-free diet until the summer of 2007 when she fairly quickly started to have pronounced symptoms. Like her sister, she started with the daily headaches and stomach aches. She was crying every day and clinging to me. She had failed to gain weight in the previous year, and was pale and thin with large, dark circles under her eyes. The paediatrician and allergist had nothing to offer, although they were concerned about her lack of weight gain. Worried that she was too sick to start second grade, I put her on a gluten-free diet. Like her sister, she improved somewhat, but did not get well. She was able to go to school, but school was now hard for her.

We were all exhausted from the lack of sleep, the worry over why our kids were so sickly, and the managing of their special diets. In November of 2007 you spoke at the Weston A. Price conference. Shortly after that all the people I knew who had attended your lectures were abuzz with what you were saying about the health of the gut, allergies, and learning. I bought your book and tapes of your lecture. Our family fit the picture perfectly, with my chronic fatigue and food allergies and all of our daughter's symptoms.

We started the GAPS Diet in late November 2007. Both of our girls were eager to try it because they felt so terrible so often. The first few months were hard, with lots of detox reactions, some improvements, and then flare-ups. The hardest part for me was worrying over every flare-up, wondering if the diet was really working, or if this, too, was going to leave us not really well. As time went on, their flare-ups became less often and less severe. Our older daughter started to gain weight. The headaches and stomach aches became rare. The crying stopped, we started sleeping at night.

I am happy to say that now, almost two years later, our couch is almost always vacant. Our girls are too busy to spend time on the couch. Our older daughter loves to horseback ride, play tennis and swim. Our younger daughter is on the soccer team, does karate, rides horses and swims. They have both needed tutoring to catch up in school, but now are both fully on grade level in all of their subjects. They are still on the GAPS diet, and we still adhere to it carefully, but we have added in a few foods slowly over the last six months, and that keeps the girls happy.

As for myself on the diet, it is taking me much longer to heal. I have seen improvements in my energy and my brain fog has mostly cleared. I still have insomnia almost every night. I still cannot include fruit or honey into my diet. I still have flare-ups and relapses of my chronic fatigue. But, I see improvements from two years ago, and from watching my girls' healing, I can see that I am on the road, I just have further to go.

To anyone who says this diet is too much work, or too hard, I reply that it is too much work and too hard to live life NOT doing the diet, living with the daily drain and worry of sick children!

Dr Natasha, I am beyond grateful to you for giving us the path to getting our children back, giving them the gift of an active healthy childhood that is every child's right!

A comment from Dr Natasha

Thank you for this story, Nancy! There are millions of families such as this in the world, where children are not really 'disabled' but are not functioning normally either. They are not healthy and do not have enough energy or enthusiasm to live their lives to the full and to enjoy the experience. Their bodies are constantly in a survival mode, 'just making it from day to day'. Should we really let our children live a life of miserable survival? Nancy is absolutely correct: every child's BIRTH RIGHT is to have a healthy and active childhood, which is followed by a healthy, happy and successful adult life. This is the choice parents, like Nancy, have made for their children. And I am sure that their children will thank them for it.

9

Melinda DeGier

Key words: autism

Our daughter Grace was diagnosed with autism on the 12th of April 2010 by Wisconsin Early Autism Project. My husband and I started to notice that something was not right with Grace shortly after we moved to Wisconsin in August of 2009. Grace was talking only in movie lines and TV lines. She could not formulate an original sentence of her own. She stared off into space a lot and had poor eye contact. She had little interest in her new baby brother and had little interest in anyone besides my husband and me. She had repetitive behaviours and liked her routines a lot.

My friend told me about the GAPS Diet and my husband and I were very sceptical and almost offended by the mentioning of a diet by a friend who did not have a child with autism. This friend finally gave us a video of Dr Natasha explaining the diet and why it works. We were astonished when we watched it. It was as though Dr Natasha was explaining Grace's health history when she was talking about her typical patients' health history. Grace had constipation issues since September of 2008 right after she had the biggest fever I ever remember her having. When she finally passed that stool, that started it all, it was like she was giving birth as she passed it. She had many ear infections treated by antibiotics shortly after her one year birthday. She had a period of time where she was pooping white stools. She had frothy stools and even had pneumonia at one point.

We started Grace on the GAPS Diet 19 June 2010. 21 June Grace seemed really out of it and I thought she must be having a lot of die-off. On 22 June in the second half of the day Grace seemed to snap out of it and she was really engaged with me. She helped me weed the

55

gardens outside our house; she played in a shallow hole with water in it all by herself and was putting leaves in it that she could find. We went inside the house and we played at her art table and she formulated a sentence properly. She said, "I have a pink marker". We had a lot of eye contact and she put her marker up in the air and said, "My marker is up high". That same day she greeted a neighbour with a "Hi" and it was spontaneous without any prompting. She did other great things that day that were all new to her!

23 June Grace was playing with her toy babies all by herself without me starting the play, which was usually what was done. She came up to me with one of her dolls and said something to the effect that the baby wants to go outside and ride the tricycle. I have never modelled this and she had never done this before! We went outside and she brought the doll and placed it on the tricycle and pushed it all around. If the doll fell she would say things like "Baby, you have to sit up!" We played with bubbles in the backyard and she was requesting bubbles up high and on the ground. She even tried to have the baby blow bubbles by putting the bubble pipe to its mouth. She laughed a lot and got really excited about a bubble that went really high. She used to be so repetitive with bubble blowing, and that day it was like she really saw what was going on and it was all new and exciting for her. I had never had so much fun playing with her!

Grace has continued to get better and better with her skills on this diet. My husband and I are so driven to continue with this diet because of the positive effect it has had on Grace. She started to be able to answer 'yes' and 'no' questions really well by 27 January 2011. 11-14 March 2011, I potty trained her when before this seemed impossible! By today I was just thinking that Grace is answering whatever questions really well. She also is able to answer questions from strangers really well too. As one of her therapists has put it "The sky is the limit for Grace"!

I hope this information has helped. I know how sceptical we were and we still have a hard time convincing people. I think they just don't want to believe it. It is a good thing that I kept a diary!

Following the GAPS Diet has changed my health and the health of my husband too: we both lost weight on the diet, my husband has energy now and his eczema is gone, I am less crabby and irritable and I do not have cramps and clotting with my periods anymore.

A comment from Dr Natasha

Thank you very much for this story, Melinda!

Thank you for the detailed description of your daughter's progress in the first few days from beginning the GAPS diet. For people who are not familiar with autism, it may not mean much that your child started playing with her toys appropriately, saying appropriate things at the appropriate moments, coming up with spontaneous comments and greetings, and looking you in the eye. But for people who know what autism is like, these small and simple things are no less than a miracle!

In less than a year Melinda and her husband have largely pulled their daughter out of the clutches of autism! I am sure that Grace is going to have a normal healthy life, demonstrating to the world that autism is curable.

10

Cara Comini

Key words: autism, dairy allergy, eczema, night terrors

To be honest I was adamantly avoiding GAPS for about three to four months after I learned that it could help my child. "Too low carb", I thought. "That is ridiculous! No grains? Who does that to a toddler?" So first we tried GFCF (gluten-free and casein-free), she was already mostly dairy-free because she got congested with milk (even raw milk).

With GFCF we saw huge, huge improvement within 48 hours. My child suddenly made eye contact, had the ability to learn, was interacting socially, and had very much improved with her balance. But sadly after about a week she started regressing, fairly quickly. I knew that GAPS was the next step, and encouraged by the initial results we got with dietary intervention, I was ready to start.

We started GAPS with the Introduction Diet, starting with chicken stock and boiled meat and vegetables, and slowly adding in more advanced foods like cooked peeled fruit, eggs, then raw pureed fruits and veggies, baked and fried meats, nuts, and cultured dairy. We progressed through the steps of the Introduction Diet waiting to make sure that new foods did not bring on a reaction. She was stuck on cooked veggies and fruit for a few months, which baffled me because I thought she was digesting those fine prior to GAPS. Her symptoms for not tolerating a food were usually night terrors, but it seems that everyone is different in this area.

I did the GAPS Introduction Diet with her. I like to try out any 'experiment' I do on my child myself, to make sure it's okay. I felt great on the diet, so I didn't worry about having her on it. I was able to progress through the stages much more quickly than she was, and I healed my dairy allergy in the process in only two months! My breastfeeding son

(11 months at this time) also went through the diet with us, and his babyhood eczema hasn't been seen again since we went on GAPS.

On 'Full GAPS' (the diet after Intro is called Full GAPS, some people only do this part of the diet and still see great success) cultured dairy is allowed. This includes 24-hour yogurt, hard cheeses and butter. After healing our initial dairy allergy (my daughter's went away quickly too, but I was nervous about trying dairy with her so I waited about four to five months) we did introduce butter, yogurt, kefir, and cheese, and we were excited about it! We kept them in for about six months and then, as a trial, I took both kids back off dairy and they started sleeping better.

As I noted above, just by reducing gluten and casein we saw a huge difference in my daughter with autism. But then she regressed. She stopped regressing within a few days of being on GAPS. For the rest of our family we see a difference within three to five days. GAPS is a very healthy 'clean' diet, and I feel like it would be a great pregnancy diet! I would just do what's called 'Full Gaps' and take it really slow introducing probiotics.

I don't stay on GAPS all the time, though I do keep my ASD child on it at all times. I anticipate that she will be on it for at least another two years (she has been on it for over a year now). The goal of GAPS is to heal the gut, and once the gut is healed non-GAPS food will be tolerated. In my case I saw this: my milk allergy went away for good, even when I was off GAPS for months.

Children often are very hungry for the first six to eight weeks on the diet; my toddler ate as much as I did the first six weeks she was on the diet. Her appetite has since calmed down; she is still a great eater, but can now go for hours between meals rather than requiring constant huge meals and snacks. The food is more nutrient-dense, and children are often less picky while on GAPS/SCD, so less food gets wasted. A common day for my four-year-old is: 2–3 eggs, scrambled + a piece of fruit for breakfast, three-five grain-free crackers or half a grain-free muffin for a snack, a palm-sized (her palm size) meat patty + a serving of lacto-fermented vegetables (1 small pickle, 1/four cup of sauerkraut) and another piece of fruit for lunch, a handful (her hand size) of nuts and dried fruit as an afternoon snack, two servings of meat (palm sized) + 1/two cup cooked veggies + 1/two cup squash fries (cooked in coconut oil) for dinner.

I personally have found GAPS to be weight normalizing – i.e. my children gain steadily (as they should!) on GAPS, while I lost a certain amount and then held there. For me that is about 135 lb at 5'8", which is my healthy weight. I personally do not watch my carbohydrate intake at all; I easily will eat four-five pieces of fruit + honey as a sweetener as often as I desire on GAPS. I have had issues with hypoglycaemia my whole life, and that is never an issue on GAPS, even without limiting my carbs.

You can learn more on Cara's website healthhomehappy.com

A comment from Dr Natasha

Thank you, Cara, for this story and your very informative website! There are many people in the world, who are dealing with the same health problems, and your thoughts and observations are very valuable for them. You came to the same conclusion many other parents of autistic children have had to come to: GFCF diet does not heal the gut and does not address the real cause of autism. Yes, removing two groups of toxins out of the body (from casein and gluten) can bring an initial improvement, but it is not enough to heal the child.

11

Kris Gustafson

BA, NTP, CHFS, Certified GAPS Practitioner

Key words: digestive problems, anxiety, hyperactivity, autistic spectrum disorder, eczema, fatigue, recurrent ear infections, migraines, constipation

Our GAPS Journey

Growing up, I could hardly wait to be a mom and have children. On the way towards that goal, I fulfilled my dream of teaching at elementary school, married a wonderful and supportive husband, and I was looking forward to having kids so that I could feed them hot dogs and Kool-Aid on warm summer days. Life was going to be good. Our first child, a girl, arrived in 1997. She quickly challenged our sanity with three months of colic, and another six months of severe constipation. But then she got 'better'. We thought that our life as parents would be smooth sailing from then on. Little did we realize the magnitude of the storm that was still to come!

Our second child, a boy, was born two and a half years later. At two weeks old, he cried 18 hours a day due to severe abdominal pain. It was only after seeing four medical doctors that we found one who suggested that our son could be reacting to my breast milk. Indeed, he was, and he was put on a very expensive 'designer' soy formula. He had severe constipation and was given daily suppositories along with a prescription to keep him regular. My mom, husband, and I each took four-hour shifts holding and rocking him around the clock for many months. The multiple paediatricians and specialists we went to could not figure out anything physically wrong with him. One doctor put him on high doses of Karo Syrup (pure high fructose corn syrup) for his

61

constipation. He had every test imaginable (most of them very invasive), each one leaving us with no answers. In desperation, I asked our state's top paediatric gastroenterologist, "If he were *your* child where would *you* go from here?" He simply shrugged his shoulders and sighed, "I have no idea". I whispered, "Then we are done". I could hardly drive home through the tears. By now (at about 18 months) my son's immune system was taking a turn for the worse. His ear infections were becoming chronic and each time he was prescribed a stronger antibiotic. He eventually ended up with tubes in his ears. But things were going to get worse. A lot worse!

At this time he started to exhibit unusual behaviours (three months after his first MMR vaccination, interestingly enough). His tantrums were frequent and lasted longer than the 'typical two-year-old'. He would hit me up to 200 times a day, leaving bruises on my legs and arms. He made constant noises with his mouth and constantly craved pressure against his body. Whenever he would stand next to me he would press so hard with his body I would lose my balance. He began exhibiting repetitive actions such as kicking walls and touching someone's face over and over again. He also had adverse reactions to strong sounds and smells. He would wear shorts in the winter and sweatpants in the summer. When he was a little older he began to leapfrog around the house. Through all of this, I could tell by looking into his eyes that he was suffering inside too. This little boy had an internal 'engine' that would not shut off. His mind and body were constantly in a state of anxiety. I knew something was not right, but the paediatrician said he was too young for any sort of diagnosis. Each night I would cry myself to sleep. I HAD to find some answers. I WOULD find some answers. I was his mother! Thus began my long and lonely journey.

Then one day, while in a bookstore, I came across a book titled, *The Sensory Sensitive Child* by Karen A. Smith, Ph, and Karen R. Gouze, PhD. I sat down on the floor and opened the book. I immediately knew they were talking about my son! Tears began to stream down my cheeks and since they splashed on the pages of the book I knew I was destined to purchase it. Now I knew *what* was wrong with him, but I had few accurate ideas about what to *do* about it. Our confusion and tribulation would continue for three more years before I would find the answers we were looking for.

My son's diet was already what I *thought* was 'dairy-free,' but then I began to learn about casein and whey (I wish I had known about this while breastfeeding!). After educating myself on dairy, gluten was removed next. Removing these two things from his diet provided some improvement, but it was not enough. His symptoms seemed to be multiplying. By this time he had been diagnosed with Sensory Processing Disorder and was exhibiting a number of other behaviours: hyperactivity, obsessive compulsive behaviour (OCD), tics, severe anxiety, anger, self-destructive behaviour, and night terrors. He was seeing a children's psychologist for the anxiety and an occupational therapist for his sensory processing. And then, our challenges were about to increase. I was pregnant again.

Our third child, another little girl, was a wonderful, healthy baby until we started to feed her baby cereal around six months of age. Her pain and constipation were so severe we were taking her to the emergency room! Could our life be any more complicated? In desperation, we went to a recommended chiropractor. Having grown up with traditional Western medicine, we did not know what to expect and were a bit sceptical. But he helped our daughter's constipation problem within a week by using magnesium.

He had an audience.

He suggested having some lab work done on her (and subsequently our son, then age seven). Their blood work showed many food intolerances. To our surprise our son showed a high reaction to almost every possible grain, many we had never heard of before, such as quinoa and amaranth. Ah-ha! *Food* sensitivities and something called 'leaky gut' as well as mild ulcerative colitis. Leaky gut occurs when the digestive system is compromised to a point where individuals are not breaking down their proteins in the stomach, so the gut becomes too permeable. The proteins begin crossing the GI barrier into the blood stream, inappropriately, and our body creates an antibody in response and the proteins now become an antigen.

We ended up taking our son of all grains and other offending foods for three months, but again, only noticed slight improvement. What I did not realize was that we were missing the mark. Gluten free/casein free was not enough, nor was being grain free. I had pieces of the puzzle, but I still did not have the whole picture. While working at our food co-op in customer service I began noticing the number of individuals coming in with food sensitivities. I was well known as the go-to person throughout our store, because I had two children with limited diets as well. As I read more and more labels, I came to realize that all I was giving the customers was the same pre-packaged junk from the conventional grocery stores, only organic, and perhaps a little healthier. A light bulb came on for me. It was all about the *food*. Our bodies need nourishing foods, not prepackaged foods with the offending allergens taken out!

I reasoned that if I was actually going to wrap my mind around all of this I needed an education in nutrition, but not just *any* nutrition. A co-worker at the co-op told me about a programme through the Nutritional Therapy Association. The next day I spent time pouring over the website and contacting the NTA office. The registration deadline was in three days. It was an absolute whirlwind. How would I find time to study? How would we afford this? But I knew that I needed this course (and so did my son). In the next 48 hours I was registered for the next class, and reading about my first NTA conference.

The conference was entitled: 'Thinking about Food: Nutrition and Mental Health'. After learning more about one of the speakers, Dr Natasha Campbell-McBride, I knew I had to go. I had never heard about Dr Campbell-McBride or her Gut And Psychology Syndrome (GAPS) diet, but she would change our lives in ways we would never have imagined. The diet removes all grains and offending sugars to heal digestive disorders. Her diet heavily focuses on the benefits of fermented dairy and vegetables, healing bone broths, and only freshly pressed juices for natural detoxification. Hearing Dr Campbell-McBride was such a privilege. Having had an autistic child she understood what it was like to truly be an advocate for her child and never giving up until she found answers. As a neurologist, with a master's degree in nutrition, she unveiled the connection between what we eat, the state of the digestive system, and learning disabilities. She was warm, kind and humble. Her message and knowledge gave me hope, and finally - a plan.

The next six months were dedicated to my studies as a NTA student, and reading as much as I could about the GAPS diet. After graduating from the NTA programme I had the time to implement the diet with our family. Before starting the diet in earnest we went on a modified version of the Full GAPS Diet. I am pleased that we did, because even with the modified version we experienced some die-off. After a couple of months we were ready to begin the Introduction Diet. Each stage gradually added in new foods, so we could easily see if one of us was reacting to something. It was one of the most challenging things we have done as a family. There were tears and laughter, resentment and forgiveness, and a lot of time as a family in the kitchen. However, it was a year's worth of healing that we would not trade for the world!

My three-year old daughter's severe constipation cleared up completely, her eczema cleared up by 90%, and her fatigue disappeared. My 12-year-old daughter's *candida* (with minimal supplementation) went away, as well as her adrenal fatigue, which she had been experiencing for years. My son, 10 at the time, had no more night terrors, his anxiety was all but gone, and his energy was that of a 'normal' 10-year-old boy. He discontinued his psychological and occupational therapy. The psychologist said, "This is clearly biological", and asked for my business cards after I graduated from the NTA programme. The occupational therapist said, "Whatever you are doing is working. I would rather have you spend your time in the kitchen for your son rather than spend two hours a week bringing him here!"

We are in our second year of the GAPS Programme and are committed to the two year minimum and beyond. We have seen great results in our children, and my chronic migraines of 30 years are almost gone. But our biggest success has been to truly have our son returned to us. He is calmer, happier, and has a wonderful sense of humour. He once told me, 'It used to feel like things were crawling all over inside my body and I couldn't make it stop.' I think *any* of us would exhibit very different behaviour if we felt something similar. He is very good at sports, has progressed through many belts in karate, and has won multiple first place trophies. He is a very bright and tenderhearted child and well liked by his peers.

Dr Campbell-McBride claims that the following conditions can significantly improve or be alleviated by using the GAPS Nutritional Protocol: autism, dyslexia, depression, dyspraxia, ADD, ADHD, schizophrenia, etc. Many of these GAPS individuals have severely impaired digestive systems. The purpose of the diet is to heal the digestive tract while repopulating with beneficial bacteria.

Because my passion has always been with children, my practice is steadily growing with paediatric clients and their families, which undoubtedly include severely compromised digestive systems. My heart breaks when I see parents screaming at their kids in frustration as they bounce off the walls, and then giving them the very toxin to snack on that is contributing to the problem. It is extremely rewarding to educate families towards hope and healing and it is never a one-size-fits-all protocol. Our journey is still not without trials, but it is through these times that we grow the most. My goal is to help others who may be experiencing the turmoil associated with families who are suffering from compromised health; to let them know that they do not need to do this alone. Everyone deserves a chance! My intention is to offer help and hope to as many as I can!

A comment from Dr Natasha

Thank you, Kris, for this wonderful story!

Kris has a beautiful family, which keeps her very busy. Nevertheless she finds time to help others: following her education with NTA Chris has certified as a GAPS Practitioner in the autumn 2011, and has a busy practice.

12

Denise

Key words: autism, adopted children, epileptic seizures

Rebirth
(translated from French)

January 2007

This is the story of our eldest son.

With this evidence, you will realize the effectiveness of the treatment that Dr Natasha Campbell-Mcbride proposes.

We adopted our son when he was only five months old.

Born prematurely, he stayed for two months in a modern unit for premature babies. When he left, he had no health problems and had a good weight. A nurse wrote in his file "very intelligent child, advanced for his age". During those two months, he nevertheless received a lot of antibiotics. Then from three to five months of age he lived in an orphanage where the medical and emotional framework was inadequate. Immediately, he showed signs of decompensation and started to vomit, he lost weight, caught a lot of viral and bacterial infections and constantly received two different antibiotics; during these three months he became withdrawn and reacted to the environment less and less.

As soon as we started to take care of him, our son came alive; he started to smile and tried to move a little on his cover. An anti-reflux drug was prescribed to prevent the mounting acid in his stomach from burning his oesophagus and giving him too much pain. After this treatment and after changing the milk, the vomiting abated. A health assessment was made on our arrival in Switzerland. It showed a series of imbalances: oesophagitis, gastro-oesophageal reflux, significant anaemia, liver too large, IgE 50 times above the norm (IgEs are proteins that play a key role in defending the body against attacks).

Up to the age of two and a half our son developed normally, but had severe physical health problems requiring constant consultations, hospitals, a multitude of drugs and surgery. He had a chronic cold, a continuous chesty cough and spastic bronchitis; he often suffered from ear infections, sinusitis, abdominal pain and had almost constant foul-smelling diarrhoea; his tonsils were permanently enlarged, he had peak 40°C (104°F) fever on and off without other symptoms, was intolerant to bovine protein, and he had a grand-mal epileptic fit.

For all these symptoms, he received nasal drops, cough mixtures, expectorants, painkillers, anti-inflammatories, antibiotics, bronchodilator sprays (Ventolin), corticosteroid sprays (Axotide), antacids (Riopan and Ulcogant), antivomitives (Primperan), gastric motility

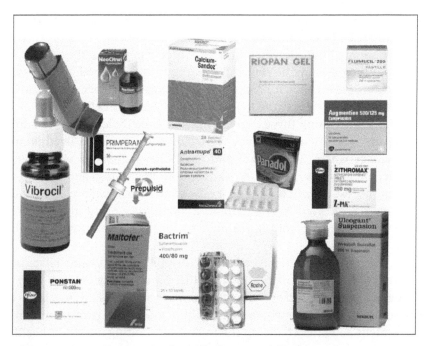

Figure 1: Drugs prescribed until change of diet

stimulants (Prepulsid) a proton pump inhibitor to block the secretion of stomach acid (Antra MUPS).

At two and a half, he received the MMR vaccine.

From that point on the situation immediately worsened and he developed confusing symptoms (physical and behavioural disorders). His gastro-oesophageal reflux, which had been more or less stabilized, came back. To treat his reflux our son had a stomach operation in July 2003; he was then three and a half years old. I thought we were beginning to see the light at the end of the tunnel and that this operation would put an end to his suffering. But shortly after the operation, I was disillusioned: reflux had not diminished and he was worse physically and mentally than before.

Here are the symptoms he presented at that time:

Physical symptoms	Mental symptoms
• gastro-oesophageal reflux	• trouble getting to sleep
• abdominal pain	• rejection of physical contact
• need to spit frequently	• hypersensitivity to smells
• digestive transit disorder	• huge sensitivity to frustrations
• constant ENT problems	• fits of rage and violence
• occasional limping	• unhappy after his fits
• pain in his feet and arms	• difficulty in respecting imposed
• unable to walk when in	limit
pain	• difficulty in being quiet at any
• stomach bloated and	time, cannot remain still
tender	• eats little at a time
• considerable night sweats	• annoying children who come to
• frequent nosebleeds	the house
• sticky eyes in the morning	• inability to play alone, cannot
• blood in stools	remain alone in a room
• excessive thirst	• very agitated or stays under
• dark circles under the eyes	a blanket on the couch
• brittle, broken and	• intense fear all the time
ingrown nails	• cannot go upstairs alone
• severe headaches	• unable to go outside alone

Physical symptoms	Mental symptoms
• agitated when his bladder full	• follows me everywhere
• burning sensation during urination	• crying a lot
• urine sometimes thick and whitish	• hypersensitive
• IgE increased dramatically	• separation very difficult
• low iron status	• permanent state of stress
• superficial breathing	• greater agitation after general anaesthetic
• poor stamina and strength	
• impetigo at four years old	

The numerous medical consultations were unbearable because I was not listened to, not taken seriously, but was considered as an over-anxious mother. After a final consultation at the hospital I decided to take another direction. I spent my evenings and my nights on the Internet doing research and filling files; during the day I contacted the people whose publications I had read.

My child was suffering greatly and we had to find a solution to help him. The sentence written in his medical records in neonatology "smart child, advanced for his age" continued to haunt me. Despite the symptoms, there were times when he was affectionate, when he thought about others, when he showed great intelligence and creativity, was reasonable and cuddled his sister.

The first thing I tried was the Kousmine Diet (a vegetarian diet based on whole grains and cold pressed oils). I emptied my cupboards to the delight of my housekeeper. (Figure 2)

Our son calmed down a bit, but still had pains in his stomach.

Six months later, I began the Herta Hafer Diet without phosphates (German chemist). Progress continued, but he still had stomach pains. Two months later, I again emptied my cupboards (again to the delight of my housekeeper) and set up the 'gluten and casein-free' diet. This

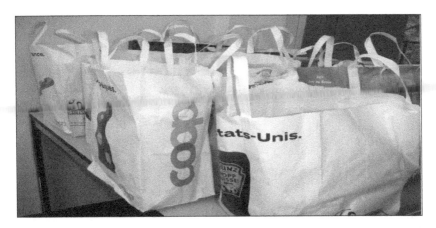

Figure 2: Foods I removed from the house when starting the Kousmine Diet

was in July 2004. Then, our son started to change: he became more peaceful, the stomach pains decreased. In three weeks, all the drugs which he had been given daily since he was a baby were stopped without relapse. He started kindergarten at the end of August 2004. The teacher was full of compliments about my son's behaviour. I thought I had won my bet: that his health problems would be resolved before starting school.

Little by little, I got used to this new cooking and cooked more and more quinoa (gluten-free cereal) and potatoes. Six months later – relapse: our son had again great stomach pains, acute gastritis and his behaviour deteriorated again. I continued my research and removed all cereals. It was then that I discovered the book by Dr Campbell-McBride *Gut and Psychology Syndrome*. This was my reading in the summer of 2005. Convinced by her theory, I began to review the content of my meals in August 2005: I reduced sugars allowed in the previous diets and gradually removed all starches. In October 2005 I met Dr Campbell-McBride in England and this was the beginning of the serious diet.

Here's what our son sent to Dr Campbell-McBride after a month and a half of her diet:

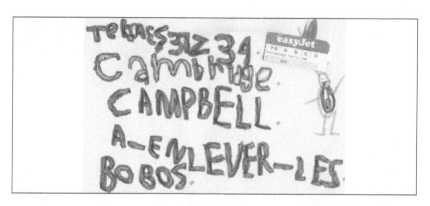

Figure 3: Drawing after a month of the GAPS Diet (translation: "flight to Cambridge, Campbell, to relieve the pain").

By the eleventh month of strict diet we had the impression of living a miracle. Our son had no more stomach ache and he slept 11 hours at a time each night without waking up. He was cooperative, played a lot and made a lot of friends. At school he was quite gifted and wanted to succeed. Nevertheless he remained very sensitive to changes of places, people, materials and food. Not all foods allowed in the plan had been introduced yet, but it was only a matter of time.

We were extremely lucky: our son had great potential and was very intelligent. He could always explain, since he was very young, what was wrong and where he was hurting. He could also express his mental problems in words or in a drawing.

Here's the kind of drawing he did when he was very afraid and was prone to fits of violence:

Afterwards, he did not dare to look at his drawings again because they terrified him. At these moments he said that he would like to remove his head, because in it there were things that were too scary.

Before October 2005 one evening he said to me "Mom, you will never find out why I have stomach aches", and he listed all the doctors and therapists who had not been able to find a solution. This statement motivated me to continue my research. And we eventually got it!

Through his intelligence and his experience our son cooperated fully and did not break his diet. The whole family went on the GAPS

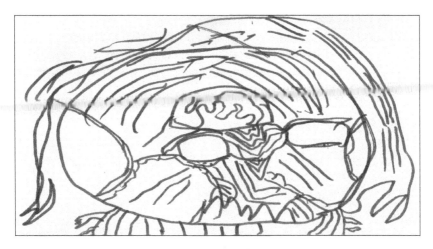

Figure 4: Drawing in a period of 'fear'.

diet. Thanks to my son, who made us change our diet, each member of our family has experienced a small miracle:

- My husband got rid of his hay fever which had plagued him for 20 years; he no longer has low morale, lost 20 kg and has more energy than he has ever had before.
- The digestive problems that I had had since adolescence went away; my chronic cold and cough, which had accompanied me for 20 years, disappeared; the pains in my back, knees and hips are gone; my energy has come back and I do not need so many hours of sleep anymore.
- As for our daughter, that we adopted when she was five weeks old, she experienced the same miracle as her brother. She had all the symptoms of her brother, just as severe. Until the age of 12 months, she had mainly digestive disorders and repeated ear and throat infections. The MMR vaccination was done at 12 months and her state immediately worsened. Before the GAPS Diet (which she started at the age of three years) she was inactive, never played, had obsessions, did not sleep well, hardly ate anything, cried all day, wanted to be in my arms all day, had a huge language

deficit and a major problem with dyspraxia. Now she is like a ray of sunshine: she chatters happily all day, plays alone (often with her Barbie dolls, of course) and she is doing very well at school. Every day she is becoming more and more confident and sure of herself.

Finally there is the sound of laughter in our house!
We are very grateful to our children for showing us the way!
We are very grateful to Natasha Campbell-McBride for her valuable advice and encouragement.

October 2008

Our children are seven and a half and nine years old. It has been three years since we began to follow Dr N. Campbell-McBride's recommendations. Now for nearly four months our two children have been stable and no longer present any health problems! They continue to take probiotics and fish oils every day; no deviation from the GAPS diet, but many new foods have been introduced. Before reaching this balance, our son had all possible complications imaginable: intolerance to foods and food supplements, fainting episodes and frequent 'die-off' reactions. We tried many foods and supplements before finally managing to stabilize the situation.

Now our two children have developed a great friendship and play a lot together. They have good aptitude at school, and our house is always filled with friends, laughter, apple tarts and almond pancakes that everybody loves! Reading this again, I realize once more the miracles that have happened; miracles which demanded so much work. But what a reward!

Dr Natasha was our 'good fairy'; we will always be grateful to her ...

A comment from Dr Natasha

Thank you, Denise, for this wonderful story!

Denis has beautiful children who continue thriving. Her son had more challenges on the way, but with his determination and Denise's help I have no doubt that all challenges will be overcome. Denise has trained as a Certified GAPS Practitioner and is helping many families in French-speaking countries. Her clients are very fortunate: they work with a practitioner who has had a personal experience of dealing successfully with a huge number of health problems!

13

Dawn Wiley

Key words: epilepsy, Dravet syndrome (a form of childhood epilepsy), prolonged use of antibiotics, kidney reflux

Kennedy May Willey was born into this world on Thursday, 13 March at 3:38a.m. She was born with kidney reflux and was started on antibiotics the day she was born. This may or may not be the point when the problems started, but I believe it is. Within three weeks of starting this medication, she started getting a really bad case of baby acne. I was told this was normal. I now believe this is not normal and this was the first sign her little body was giving that her immune system was being suppressed by the antibiotics and was on toxic overload.

At her two-month check-up, she was given her two-month vaccinations and was put on heavier duty antibiotics. At four months, she was given yet more vaccinations but was told she could go off the antibiotics. As soon as she was taken off the antibiotics she stopped sleeping through the night and immediately developed acid reflux, yet another sign that her body was not operating at its full potential.

Within two months, the ear infections started and we went back on antibiotics. She had four ear infections in three months.

'Antibiotics have a direct damaging effect on the immune system, making one more vulnerable to infections, which leads to a vicious cycle of more antibiotics and more infections' – *Gut And Psychology Syndrome*, Dr Natasha Campbell-McBride MD.

So here we were in our ever-present cycle of infections and digestive issues (i.e. reflux) and we continued vaccinating an unhealthy child.

'The manufacturers of vaccines produce them for children with normal immune systems which will react to these vaccines in a predictable way. However, in modern society with our modern way of life, we are rapidly moving to a situation where a growing proportion of children do not have a normal immune system and will not produce expected reaction to the vaccine. In some of these children vaccination becomes that 'last straw which breaks the camel's back' and brings on the beginning of epilepsy. It is the state of the child's immune system that appears to be the decisive factor, not the vaccines' – *Gut And Psychology Syndrome*, Dr Natasha Campbell-McBride, MD.

On 26 December 2008 within eight days of receiving her DPT vaccination, Kennedy suffered a 40-minute seizure. Three years later and with a diagnosis of Dravet syndrome, Kennedy has had 63 seizures. Medication was the only answer we received from countless doctors and we tried it after she had five seizures in one day. However, when she was on medication she was lethargic and lifeless and I couldn't bear to see her like that. My husband and I decided we would rather deal with the seizures.

We sought alternative treatments for Kennedy and every time we did she would have a span of months with no seizure activity. Finally, after visiting the top specialist in the U.S. in regards to Dravet and her only answer being a cocktail of three medications, we completely put our trust into alternative therapies. We took many different approaches, but the one that finally worked was the one I put off time and time again. The diet is called the GAPS Diet and it is directly based on the SCD diet. I read as much as I could in one night of Dr Campbell-McBride's website and then immediately ordered her book *Gut And Psychology Syndrome*. I engulfed her book in less than a week and then turned around and finally read *Breaking the Vicious Cycle* by Elaine Gottschall. The reason I hadn't been interested in Elaine's book is because she doesn't really address epilepsy, so I really thought it had nothing to do with us. But the recently released new edition of the *Gut And Psychology* book has an epilepsy chapter in it. I was hooked. Pieces started to come together. Things were starting to make a little sense.

On 17 March 2011, we started the SCD diet for Kennedy. Within a couple months we transitioned over to the GAPS Diet. Our life has dramatically changed since starting this nutritional journey for Kennedy. Kennedy used to seize at least once a week. Her seizures were triggered by all kinds of things; sometimes we didn't even know the trigger. The biggest triggers were illness, heat and exhaustion. Now her seizures have cut down to almost nil. It is truly a miracle!

Kennedy had a terrible immune system. Her allergies were constant and we were guaranteed respiratory infections at least once a year. The allergies quit the minute we started the diet, and any illness she has contracted within the last year has been short and gone within a day. This is one of the biggest changes we have seen in Kennedy.

Kennedy could not do anything outside that raised her temperature even a little bit. This past year and one month Kennedy has not had one seizure relative to heat. She joined the cheer team, the soccer team, horseback riding lessons and is able to participate in all outdoor fun and activities. For the first time in her short little life, she has been able to fully experience the joy of being a kid.

This has not been an easy road and we have had to go against a lot of mainstream recommendations to get to this place. One of the most controversial decisions we have had to make was NOT putting Kennedy on anti-epileptic drugs. I know that this is one of the main reasons that she is doing as well as she is today. Now Kennedy is a completely normal child!

A comment from Dr Natasha

Children with Dravet syndrome usually have a poor response to anti-epileptic medication and poor prognoses: they are expected to have impaired mental and physical development. Little Kennedy May is developing normally and living a very happy busy life!

Dawn Wiley runs a website with regular updates on Kennedy's health, homefoodheals.com, where you can see videos with this beautiful little girl doing all the normal things children of her age do. Thank you for this wonderful work, Dawn, and for allowing the world to learn from your experience!

14

Sonia Zukoski

Key words: autism / PDD (Pervasive Developmental Disorder), fussy eating, recurrent ear infections, antibiotics

My name is Sonia. My husband and I are parents of two beautiful children: Jennifer, who is 11 years old and Nicholas, five years old. I was raised in Brazil and my husband is from the US; neither of our families had any record of childhood abnormalities.

Jennifer was born six weeks early but reached all her milestones at the right time. Five years after Jennifer was born we had a boy. Nicholas was born full-term. Up until his birth (in 2006) I had no idea what autism was.

I breastfed Nicholas for five months and, although he was a bit fussy, everything was going well. He started talking around one year of age. He was a very happy kid, very involved and just a joy. Around eighteen months however Nicholas started regressing. He started to get ear infections one after another and with that came antibiotics one after another. I saw the negative effects of those drugs and started doing the research on my own for natural remedies. The ENT (ear, nose and throat) specialist recommended putting saline drops into Nicholas' nose three times a day to stop ear infections. I tried that for one month without effect, and the doctor proposed putting ear tubes in (grommets). I left the doctor's office determined that my son would not get ear tubes. I read that equal parts of alcohol and vinegar used as drops in the ear would dry the water in the ear and kill the bacteria; I started using that. To build his immune system I started feeding him three full syringes (three times a day) of blended and strained raw fruits and vegetables with fish oil added and Echinacea. I was just praying that this blend of raw fruits and vegetables would work. And it did.

One month later the ENT doctor said that Nicholas did not need ear tubes! I was so happy from that point; now Nicholas didn't need any more antibiotics or over-the-counter medication for infections.

Nevertheless Nicholas continued to regress: not talking anymore, not making eye contact and, worst of all, not eating. He would only eat bananas, pizza and any kind of bread with peanut butter. I continued giving him blended raw fruits and vegetables, as I knew my son was not getting enough nutrients.

Soon, Nicholas was diagnosed with autism/PDD. We could not afford to go to a DAN doctor because they are so expensive. Besides, I had heard about so many different treatments for autism; it was very confusing where to begin. Every day I hoped to come across something that would help my son! It was around July 2011 that I heard about the book *Gut and Psychology Syndrome* by Dr Natasha Campbell-McBride. I read the book, and in August 2011 I started Nicholas on the Full GAPS Diet, and one month later I started him on the GAPS Intro.

The first plate of soup was a real nightmare: Nicholas kicked me, bit me, screamed, and pulled my hair. It took me three hours to feed him one bowl of soup! I could not bribe him with anything. It was a session of horror for him and for me! The second day it took me 45 minutes to feed him a bowl of soup. Little by little I was able to bribe him to eat the soup. It was heart-breaking to see him begging for bananas and pizza and having to say no. Today, after five months of the Intro Nicholas eats the soup (watching his favourite TV shows or playing educational games on the computer) without struggle. His eating disorder is disappearing little by little. Without any bribes he is eating chicken, home-made sausages, apples, pears, and all the baked goods that are allowed on stage six of the diet. Occasionally he gets fussy and becomes a picky eater again, due to die-off.

We started to see improvements in his behaviour: Nicholas does not jump up and down anymore and doesn't run away like he used to. His tantrums are a lot less than they used to be prior to the diet. I know that Nicholas is far from being healed from autism yet, but I'm very thankful to Dr Natasha for her book. This book gives us a chance of helping our children, who are suffering from a condition that is considered to have no cure in the conventional medicine! Our complete journey in healing Nicholas has a way to go yet, but I am writing a book to describe all of our challenges, and to encourage other parents. I'll publish the book sometime in 2013 or 2014. I know that without the GAPS Diet my son's story would have had a very different outcome.

A comment from Dr Natasha

Thank you, Sonia, for your story! Fussy eating is a typical symptom of GAPS conditions (such as autism). Sonia has demonstrated that this problem can be overcome, despite the fact that it can be very difficult at the beginning. The older the child is, when you start, the more difficult it is. We will all wait for Sonia's book to come out. I am sure that with Sonia's determination Nicholas will do well!

15

Lynne M. George

Key words: autism

My grandson Brandon was diagnosed with autism at the age of 17 months. When Brandon was five years old, we were told to read Dr Natasha's *Gut and Psychology Syndrome* book. GAPS empowered our family with the knowledge that most autistic individuals have inflamed guts which lead to inflamed brains. The focus of the natural treatment of GAPS is to HEAL the inflammation in the brain and the rest of the body, allowing the body to begin HEALING itself.

We follow the GAPS Diet to a 'T'. We have tested and found that any deviation from this diet causes Brandon to have a negative reaction and reversal in his progress. We have created tasty recipes for Brandon, such as pizzas (crust made from grinding almonds to a powder consistency), cookies, beetroot lemonade, fruit smoothies, breakfast juices, etc.

Along with the diet for the first two and a half years of Brandon's journey we used Bio-Kult, a probiotic created by Dr Natasha. Bio-Kult aided in healing his gut.

An important part of the treatment is reduction in Brandon's general toxic load. Dr Natasha lists everything we needed to know and gives us all the information in her GAPS book (chapter on detoxification in particular).

Dr Natasha's book *Gut and Psychology Syndrome* teaches, targets, empowers and equips us with the knowledge of natural treatments for autism. GAPS is our reference book in combating Brandon's autism, our family owns several copies.

Seeing is believing! For more information about Brandon and GAPS, go to www.brandonswindow.com and get direct links and videos of my grandson's amazing progress of reversing autism naturally. Our plight is to help others! We Are Reversing the Symptoms of Autism Using Natural Treatments!

Dr Natasha, Thank You for allowing God to use you as his tool in giving us our Brandon back!

May God Continue to Bless You and Your Family!

A comment from Dr Natasha

Lynne is a tireless campaigner for natural approaches to treating autism. Her website www.brandonswindow.com is a detailed record of her grandson's progress. It is an excellent record for anybody who wants to study autism and find an effective treatment for it. Thank you, Lynne, for this valuable work!

16

Susanna

Key words: PDD-NOS (Pervasive Developmental Disorder – Not
Otherwise Specified, this diagnosis is often given to non-typical autistic
children), lead poisoning, twins, fussy eating, food intolerances

After a very relaxed and complication-free pregnancy our twins were
born at 38 weeks gestation. Ben was born first with 2600grams, 52 cm
and 9/10 Apgar. A minute later, Julia followed with 2650 grams, 50 cm
and 9/10 Apgar score.

At the earliest age everything was splendid. The kids ate non-stop
and grew at an admirable rate. They were fed a mixed diet of mother's
milk, collected women's milk and formula. By the time they were six
months old, they had easily caught up to an 'average singleton' in all
aspects. We had to deal with a bit of infant colic and bad teething
issues, but who doesn't? Ben was hard to get on dairy products around
12 months of age, but eventually it was OK.

We lead a very busy life. They were in baby classes from the age
of three months, getting closer to full time from 18 months. Not
just because they are my kids, but Ben and Julia were doing much
better than their peers. However, even though the kids continued
to grow at a singleton rate, feeding started to become a bad experience. Finicky doesn't even describe our 18-month-old twins. We
routinely darkened the room, had a kid movie on and fed them on
the sly.

Ben has experienced really bad terrible-twos. Looking back, he may
have had some (autistic) spectrum issues, but we did not know to look
for signs. On the other hand, two kids who routinely work together to
get what they want – any parent can easily feel outnumbered. As per
developmental measures, both kids were doing wonderfully on all

scores: movement, speech and social. We were especially happy with their language development, as our family is bilingual.

Things started to go wrong when they received their tick bite shots at the age of two and a half. It was really bad timing for Ben, as he had just fallen off our terrace and had a major head trauma. Within a week we lost our baby boy. As the last attempt, he tried to talk to Julia in their special twin language. Although she understood him, she would not reply. So he shut himself off from the world.

It became blatantly obvious that Ben would not 'grow out' of the shock, or whatever it was, by the time they started formal school at age three. He was distant, self-stimulating and most noticeably: speechless. His teachers complained about lack of cooperation and respect for others. After six months on the waiting list and in hope that this whole thing would go away somehow, we received the diagnosis of PDD-NOS. Needless to say, that was a dark moment in our family's life.

By pure chance, I sat next to a paediatric gastroenterologist at a musical premiere. She urged me to bring Ben by her office. Apparently, a lot of her patients that have ASD (Autistic Spectrum Disorder) diagnosis are also suffering from food intolerance and various gastrointestinal issues. Even though Ben had not shown typical allergy signs, such as diarrhoea and spots around his mouth or on other parts of his body, I took him to see her.

To our great surprise, his casein intolerance was off the charts. When we removed casein, we saw an amazing change. It started with 10 days of horrible withdrawal symptoms: never-before-seen anger and aggressive behaviour. After that, blue skies were in store. Ben started singing rock songs and reciting full nursery rhymes. His pronunciation would be sluggish at best, but finally he started to talk again! Next he tested positive for fructose, gluten, yeast, egg-white, soy (although he never had any), several seafood items and some miscellaneous others. Slowly we removed every IgG ingredient, but we did not see great improvements. We also started any therapy that seemed promising at all: movement, horseback riding, floor-time, son-rise...etc. I am sure these may work for others, but they did not work for us.

So we decided to go to America. We got in contact with a renowned DAN! doctor, Dr Kotsanins, in Texas, who thoroughly examined Ben. The findings were shocking:

- His gut lining was severely damaged, good flora being scarce;
- Yeast and other parasites were present in staggering amounts;
- He was suffering from malnutrition and was deficient in several vitamins and minerals;
- He was lead poisoned. Ben's heavy metal burden was high, but for lead, he was over 10 times the 'approved' limit, showing significantly elevated levels of serum lead.

For the fortunate ones, who do not know anything about lead poisoning, let me elaborate a little. Any sign of lead poisoning in the blood (serum lead) is very rare. Even if one should swallow 10 fishing leads or a lead soldier, it quickly moves into the cells and is undetectable in the blood sample after a mere two to three weeks. Ben had to accrue substantial quantities of lead regularly to show such bad results. As it later turned out, it was from our tap water. We live in a 200-year-old building and some of the piping is at least a century old. Before the 60s, standard pipes were made out of lead. On a side note: every single pipe in the building has since been updated, involving all 48 flats.

Our DAN! doctor wanted to attack the lead situation, but with such a damaged gut, underperforming liver and an obviously sick little body he could not. First he had to make sure a proper diet was in place. Dr Kotsanis suggested SCD or something better: GAPS. I had heard of GAPS from fellow moms and the great things it has done for their children, so we set out to do GAPS.

My husband and Ben started GAPS Intro at the same time, following Ben's pace. This was to have a better understanding what Ben feels and how the diet affects him. My poor husband went from cinnamon rolls one morning to broth the other. I had a very grouchy husband for a few weeks.

We got through the Intro at a fairly good rate. Still, my skinny little boy lost 2 kg on the spot. This was the point when my Mom tried to intervene, and for the first time I said 'No' to my Mother. Soon, to everyone's great relief, he quickly put some weight back on and was as energetic as ever. He started to try and sometimes even eat new foods. It may sound funny, but food became interesting as opposed to outright evil. Would he want to have his GF pasta? Off course, but he was willing to try vegetables and different textures too. Soon enough, GAPS food became the norm and new food less threatening.

After four months of GAPS diet, supplementation, yeast killing and general liver build-up period, we started DMSA chelation. The protocol called for three days chelation, four days off. To be on the safe side, we have increased the off days to seven or even to 12, if there were serious reactions. Our reactions were controllable, with the exception of two episodes of 12-hour plus migraine attacks, which were quite scary. These were the result of intense detoxification at one end and slow excretion at the other. We have learned to look for signs of detox block, such as dark circles under his eyes, puffy eyes, pale grey skin and sudden behaviour changes. When we see the signs, we can now help him with glutathione, citrus pectin, cranio-sacral therapy or just an Epsom salt bath. Like everything else, one needs to learn how to manage the reactions.

In the meantime, we have made sure to test Julia for heavy metal toxicity and food sensitivities. She has not shown any symptoms at all. In fact, she is our super-talkative social butterfly, empress of the playground. Still, they drank the same tea, ate the same soup, bathed in the same water. To make a long story short, she has practically the same food sensitivities – just less severe – and turned out to be lead-poisoned as well. Her lead results were somewhat less elevated, mere over five times the regulatory limit.

It was obvious that we needed to get her on the GAPS Diet too. In fact, it made my life easier, as I had to cook only two kinds of food. She took to the diet very easily and has been doing really well ever since. We have decided to use only natural chelating methods such as chlorella, spirulina, cilantro and juicing.

Since then Ben has evolved a great deal. He has strengthened physically a lot, grew over 10 cm in the last year and gained several kilos. He is not pale and grey anymore, but well-tanned and healthy looking. He has the stamina to learn at school and the energy to swim or climb trees after school. He has reached developmental milestones incredibly fast. We have a true chance of losing his diagnosis! Oh, and his lead levels went down from 50 mcg/g to 8 mcg/g in one year with GAPS and two rounds of DMSA.

Julia has been on the diet only for six months. Still, her lead level went down from 27 mcg/g to 13 mcg/g. She continues to grow, to be smart as a whip, tall and fun. She became very health-conscious, which is sort of funny at age five. She has no qualms informing classmates how it is much healthier to eat an apple than some candy. She even goes on to explain the negative side effects of excessive sugar intake on one's body.

My husband has cleansed his system and realized that dairy products did not agree with him at all. He has also lost some weight, especially from his midsection. At 40 this is no small feat; especially since all his friends sport a beer belly, while he feels young and vivacious. Even though he went back to eating 'normal' food, he tries to eat a bowl of soup every day and has decreased his unhealthy eating habits greatly.

As we cook every meal at home and shop as organically as we can, I think we have achieved a great equilibrium. No processed food at all, minimal sugar, plenty of good fat, great vegetables... this is a sure way to stay healthy too. I trust that by establishing a healthy life now, we can cure Ben and avoid issues in the future. In fact, I am already feeling like a superhero right out of my kitchen!

Now, in the summer 2012, our healing continues and we are doing great. As Ben's body got better, his cognitive functions picked up with great speed. He has gained 4 years worth of skills in one year as measured by VB-MAPP and ABLLS. My son will start kindergarten in completely general educational system with his twin sister this fall. We are not 'done' but doing great!

A comment from Dr Natasha

You are a superhero, Susanna, because every woman who takes charge of cooking for her family takes charge of her family's health, and not only physical! Thanks to the nurture you provided (out of your kitchen) now you have a beautiful healthy family!

The human body is equipped with an excellent cleansing system, called the detoxification system. When this system works well it removes all sorts of toxins which come in from outside or are generated as by-products of our own metabolism. In GAPS children and adults the sheer level of toxicity coming into the body from the gut breaks down their detoxification system, and the body starts accumulating toxins. It is obvious that Ben's detox system got broken down; as a result he accumulated much larger amounts of lead than his twin sister Julia, and this lead affected his physical and mental development. Julia was exposed to just as much lead as Ben, but because her detox system was working better, she accumulated much less lead and it did not affect her development. In fact she appeared to be healthy and was developing normally. Still, the parents made the right decision to treat her as well. GAPS Programme helps to restore the detoxification system; and as soon as it starts working, the body starts cleaning itself very efficiently.

Thank you, Susanna for this wonderful story!

17

Susan White

Key words: ADHD (Attention Deficit Hyperactivity Disorder), ME (Myalgic Encephalomyelitis) / CFS (Chronic Fatigue Syndrome), eczema, asthma, malabsorption, diarrhoea, poor immunity

"I didn't recognize him!" exclaimed my friend recently, amazed at the change in Ben.

It is almost painful for me now to watch videos of family holidays when my son was younger, playing on the beach; he was thin and pale, ribs clearly visible, hyperactive with a high-pitched voice. Our family life was dominated by the need to make sure he could get to a toilet, because of frequent bouts of diarrhoea, and the necessity to control his diet. It was a dawning nightmare from toddlerhood onwards of having to work out which foods affected him and gradually cutting them out: dairy products, whole foods, raw food, gluten and so on.

Fearfulness at night-times and difficulty getting to and staying asleep made bedtimes a continual strain. Born when I already had ME, Ben was always underweight and constantly hungry. Eczema started as soon as I was forced to wean him on to the standard cow's milk-based baby formula at three months, because I became too ill to breastfeed him. As he grew older, colds were frequent, often accompanied by asthma symptoms – wheezing, breathlessness, weakness and coughing at night. Antibiotic overuse had been implicated in the onset of my ME. So, we did everything we could to avoid Ben having to take antibiotics and steroids of any kind, knowing that there would always be side effects. We only used a low-strength hydrocortisone cream on his eczema. We increasingly researched and used natural remedies, but we came close at times to giving in to drugs!

Ben's gut problems mirrored my own, but had come far earlier in his life, probably I guess now, from a weakened immunity and an overdose of candida from my body, when he was in the womb. For me, colitis/IBS only really started with a vengeance at age 18, a few months after leaving home, when I caught first glandular fever in Belgium (and had a strong course of penicillin); and then I got an intestinal infection. I was prescribed anti-spasmodics and psyllium husks and gradually worked out what foods upset my stomach. After six months, I was just about well enough to go to university. I learned to managed the colitis and my worsening symptoms of polycystic ovary syndrome for which I had to take the pill (which I was unaware then could affect my gut flora).

Hindsight is a wonderful thing, isn't it? Now I can see all the predisposing factors were in place. At the age of 31, when I was hit by an extremely stressful year with serious illness in my close family, and a bout of flu (and the obligatory antibiotics), my strength was decimated almost overnight. I had to give up work and ME/CFS was diagnosed. My gut problems continued to worsen with bloating, nausea, diarrhoea alternating with constipation, my bowel often not moving at all for days on end. I was diagnosed with severe gut dysbiosis; fatigue, muscle pain, tinnitus, vertigo and so on were the main features of ME for me. I was mainly housebound and could only read, listen to the radio or watch TV a few minutes at a time. Reactions to food dominated my life, and eventually (after 10 years) I could only eat a handful of foods, and I had to eat them in rotation for fear of reacting more to them: chicken, white fish, quinoa, millet, carrots, green beans and soya milk. Any divergence made me too ill to cope.

Well, it makes pretty depressing reading so far, doesn't it? With a strong Christian belief in healing, it was both agonizing that I was continuing to worsen and my son had similar problems, and exciting, having the hope that things would change. The answer to our prayers came, significantly for me, on Easter weekend 2003, when a nutritionist friend encouraged me to read a book recommended to her by a lady, who apparently got better. The book, as you have probably guessed, was *Breaking the Vicious Cycle*. When I read the first few pages of Elaine Gottschall's explanation of how gut problems develop, I nearly cried. It was the first rational, scientific reasoning I had seen, which explained so much of my and my son's problems. However, the prospect of starting the diet was very daunting. But I knew deep inside that this was the answer, so I psyched myself up over a period of weeks, made preparations, and then launched myself on it!

It was the start of a wonderful new chapter in our lives. Never again would we be at the mercy of our bowels and ill health! Gradually, our diets would widen, appetites return, weight go back on and accompanying symptoms such as asthma, rhinitis, eczema, travel sickness, etc would all but disappear. The improvements didn't come overnight and there were many ups and downs, partly as I learned to 'tweak' the diet for us as individuals.

After a few days on SCD I was hit by wave after wave of what I came to recognize as die-off symptoms, as my body began to offload toxins built up over the years, and the bad bacteria and candida died off. These phases were overwhelming to start with, but began to decrease in intensity and frequency, and in between each phase I started to feel better and better, and my digestive system strengthened to be able to reintroduce foods. I have learned a lot over the years and our progress could have been faster if I had known then what I know now. However, my own health was so fragile that I had to be very cautious. I didn't start chicken soup until a year into the diet, and then even a single teaspoon of it made me very ill because of its strong anti-microbial effect on my high toxic level. I have come to recognize the soup now as fundamental to our healing! Also, I discovered that eating too much nut undermined our progress (it's very hard on the bowel and candida likes it!) At that stage, even a single drop of lemon juice made me too ill, presumably because its acid was killing off too much bad bacteria/candida in my gut. I also didn't start having the SCD yogurt for a long time and only ate fish, meat and vegetables.

After nine months, the worst of my ME fatigue and symptoms improved significantly for the first time in over a decade, and we were so amazed that we started our ADHD son on the diet, after discovering the work of Dr Campbell-McBride and consulting with her. Having learned from my experience, we gradually transitioned him to GAPS over a period of weeks rather than overnight, so his progress was smoother and the die-off phases less noticeable.

GAPS/SCD hasn't been an easy road but it has been the foundation of our healing. I believe that the diet takes a load off the digestive system to enable it to start to heal, and also relieves the immune system to enable the body to rebalance and strengthen. It is important to tailor the diet for you – i.e. don't eat something that is technically 'legal' if you know you already react to it. In time your bowel will improve and you can reintroduce foods a little at a time, as your bowel doesn't need to react so strongly to 'protect' you from the offending food – it is your friend, so work with it! Listen to your body, don't give up and keep on seeking answers.

I spent the first few years continually on the internet support groups asking questions and getting fabulous support. I couldn't have made it without my e-community! Frequently I have discovered that it was something we were eating, or eating too much of, which was hindering our progress. Not everyone tolerates yogurt for example – for us, we still only have one tablespoon a day and get on better with probiotic capsules. Others find sauerkraut, or at least the juice from it, works for them. Anything that overloads or irritates your digestive system, with its unique sensitivities, even simply eating too large portions, will make its job harder.

It's a lot of work to provide tasty food that appeals to your child, and eating away from home is rarely easy. It was easier when Ben was small; as he got older, he became more aware of what others were eating and wanted it, or was self-conscious about his 'different' food. We've been able to let him have food off the diet on and off for a few years now, but generally speaking he is still on it at home, We have also learned that we personally needed to address issues such as low stomach acid, and use supplements like glutamine and digestive enzymes to support the healing process. Liver cleansing has made another big improvement, including liver flushes, to decongest the liver and gall bladder.

Ben is now 14, and it is such a joy and relief to be able to relax more about his diet and see him looking so strong and healthy; I can't see his ribs anymore! He has a lovely clear spot-free complexion with good colour in his cheeks, unlike a lot of his pale-looking peers plagued by spots! If his health slips back a bit, then he just goes back on the SCD/GAPS 'straight and narrow' until things improve again. In the past few months he has joined a football team, something he would-n't have had the stamina for before, and he continues to perform very well academically. When he's not having GAPS food, I try to encourage the principle of 'food combining', i.e. not mixing starch with protein, and this helps too.

I used to think that full healing would mean that we could eat the 'standard Western diet' freely, but I've come to the conclusion that this isn't logical or desirable anyway. The standard Western diet is so heavily weighted with the big cash crops (wheat, sugar and milk), which most people are eating in some form at nearly every meal. It doesn't make sense to me now to overload our bodies with a handful of foods, when there is such an enormous variety of foods available to us, with their wide range of nutrients. And, actually, we really like our SCD/GAPS way of eating – the food tastes better and our diet is far wider and healthier than it ever was before!

For myself, now in 2012 the ME symptoms have not fully gone yet, and I continue to seek the final piece of the jigsaw to make it a thing of the past. I have tried breaking the diet modestly a few times but always, over time, my digestion and overall health slips back. But I have a very acceptable level of energy and feeling of wellbeing now within these boundaries. One thing I know is that I could not have got to where I am without SCD/GAPS. Try it for yourself and see!

A comment from Dr Natasha

Thank you, Susan! Susan and Ben have been on this journey for a long time and it is wonderful to see what they have achieved! Ben is a healthy teenager enjoying his life, and Susan is doing well, considering where she started.

CFS and ME are some of the most difficult conditions to treat. Everything has to be introduced gradually, slowly and patiently: foods, supplements, detoxifying baths and any other interventions. Meat stock and bone broth are essential for these people to heal; but even this healing is often too much for them and they have to start very gradually. This story shows that success is achievable, no matter how ill you are at the beginning!

18

Eileen

Key words: autism, Oppositional-Defiant Disorder, anxiety, OCD (Obsessive Compulsive Disorder), asthma, digestive problems, cyclical vomiting syndrome, reflux, large family

I am no writer, but here is our story in a few pages. It is not finished yet, but after two years of GAPS we are getting there!

The day I typed up our story (with lots of tears), my daughter, who was not functioning at all two years ago, walked in with her G1 (learners' permit) that she got all by herself! It was her 16th birthday. I didn't even know she was going to try for it. What a wonderful birthday present, to be able to do all that on her own!

But let us start from the beginning.

My husband and I have eight children from 18 to four-year-old twins, all on the GAPS diet. You might say it is difficult to cook from scratch for eight children. But, when you hear our story, you will see that it is much easier to cook for a happy family, then to deal with all the problems that were destroying our family.

Our second child, my daughter, had constipation from birth. She lost her speech after her MMR shot and had many sensory issues. A week after stopping breast feeding she got her first ear infection, and was on antibiotics many times when she was two and three. We dragged her through tons of speech and OT (occupational therapy) therapies, but life was still such a struggle for my daughter. We took her to many doctors, but all said there were no other problems, just speech and OT. I knew better! She was never in our world, could barely speak, and when she did, the words were very jumbled up.

Finally she was diagnosed with autism at age 13, with severe anxiety, OCD and depression, which manifested itself in crying all day for weeks on end. Other problems included not changing her clothes or brushing her hair, not being able to put clothes on, or go into her room, or sleep in her bed, or go to school. She would sleep with a winter coat (all zipped up with the hood pulled tightly over her face) on the hard wood floor. She could not go into bathrooms due to high anxiety. She wouldn't take a shower: if we forced the situation, it was an hour of scratching, screaming and clawing trying to get her to take a shower. We would find her urine in various containers in our house. She would not use the toilet, but run outside and poop the few times she needed to poop (she was still constipated). Taking her out to see doctors was difficult: she would run circles around people on the street and refuse to walk down certain paths and roads, all the while angrily growling at me: saying that there was nothing wrong with her and that 'I' was the problem.

We were so hopeless! My family was crumbling under the weight of the daily battles trying to get her dressed, or go to school, or have a shower. She didn't act like she was frightened, but defiantly disobedient, inflexible, strong as an ox. When she didn't get her way, or you didn't allow her to do her OCD thing (obsessions), she would get physical, forcing the issue, or grab a knife and try to cut her wrist.

In the middle of all of this were seven other children, including 18-month-old twin girls. Two of the children had constant digestive problems, reflux, stomach pain, anxiety, and chest pains. Another child had joint pains and a bad stomach. Yet another had asthma and breathing problems: they were so bad, that she had to be rushed by ambulance to hospitals to be put on steroids and antibiotics for pneumonia. We spent most of our free time going to see different doctors, who prescribed different medications, most of which didn't work or created other problems.

My oldest child Michael always had digestive issues; as a young child he vomited every evening. That gradually moved to terrible continuous vomiting episodes, which increased in duration every time they recurred. We were in and out of hospitals as each episode grew longer in duration, and dehydration was a problem. Many tests were run and no conclusions could be reached. Once, after 14 days of constant vomiting and no answers from the hospital staff, we were told by the medics that it was psychological and that he was 'faking'.

Another specialist called it 'cyclical vomiting syndrome'. With no help (just a label, and always waiting for the next vomiting episode), Michael was so weak that he would just pass out in the middle of speaking or playing. We lived waiting for the next vomiting episode to start and life to come to a halt for weeks: Michael would get so sick, and I would be sick with worry, wondering if he would survive another day! After an episode we would slowly get our child back, and then wait 'walking on egg shells' for the next episode. Finally the John Radcliffe Hospital diagnosed him with reflux. We put him on antacid medication. But after six months my son took himself off it, saying that he didn't like how the medicine made him feel. It was at that time that Michael started to lose his concentration at school and the arguing over homework began. I didn't realize, till the same thing happened with another child, that the meds to help his stomach interfered with memory and concentration! We saw the same pattern: forgetfulness, loss of concentration and not doing well at school. We dumped the stomach meds!

With my daughter, we resorted to psychiatric drugs. Prozac made sensory issues unbearable. Try having an 80 lb child hang off your waist all day long. Also the Prozac made her constipation worse. Zoloft made her OCD much worse. Desperate for help (that no one in the medical profession seemed to be able to give), I began searching online for anyone that could help with debilitating OCD. We found GAPS and ordered the book.

When I read the book *Gut and Psychology Syndrome* it read like a book of my life! When I saw the list of highly toxic things found in modern houses, I realized: that list looked just like the list I made for my daughter's school (of things that caused huge anxiety for my daughter). Bathrooms, toilets, showers, new clothing, swimming pools, new carpeting all affected her; I remember, she wouldn't go downstairs in the basement for one year, when we installed a new carpet there. What we thought was just psychosis was actually her inability to deal with chemicals, which her body could not detoxify!

I started the GAPS Diet on myself first. After one month I realized that my asthma and allergies to dust and animals were gone! I could even change the vacuum bag in the central vac canister in the garage. So I decided to try the diet with my daughter.

The first two weeks of the diet were hell. It was like a drug user getting off heavy narcotics. She was pacing the floor like a caged lion; telling me, that she was angry with her brother and that 'she thinks she was REALLY going to kill him!'. She was so angry; she said she was never so angry before. She was craving sugar: she would sneak sugar and come home sucking the honey bottle to get sugar into her.

After a few weeks on the diet I took her to the local doctor, who specializes in autism. I showed him the GAPS book and told him about the diet. He told me that it wasn't fair to put her on the diet; that she needed to have pizza and other foods, which kids of her age like. He asked her if that was what she wanted. My daughter stood up and said, "You are right! I hate this diet and I hate my mother for forcing me on this diet, but you know what I hate even more? I hate crying all day and not knowing what is wrong with me, I hate being curled up in a ball rocking back and forth! Yes, I hate this diet, but I hate those things even more!" I was speechless!.. But the doctor didn't understand what we had been through, so didn't realize what she meant! He told me to give her milk of magnesia for the constipation and sent us home.

Slowly my daughter's anxiety lessened. It was no quick fix, but like an ice sculpture left in the sun, her problems gradually began to melt away. Anytime she cheated on her diet her anxiety spiked. After two years I can still tell when she cheats on her diet: I see OCD return.

Two years later, today is my daughters 16th birthday. Her anxiety is almost non-existent! She takes responsibility for most of her own diet. I am no longer the diet police. She combs her hair and washes her face. She goes to school daily, catching a 7:30a.m. bus, fully dressed with a lunch she packed herself. My daughter is in control of her own life! When she feels anxiety she knows to take an Epsom salt bath. When she is constipated she will eat a bowl of sauerkraut. She talks to other moms that need help starting the diet with their own children. She babysits weekly for a family of seven children, one of whom is severely autistic. My daughter was just re-evaluated for autism, and has moved from being severely autistic to moderately to mildly autistic, in two years.

Just to provide some support for my daughter we put the rest of the family on the GAPS Diet for a few weeks, and to our astonishment all their symptoms disappeared too! After two weeks on the diet, reflux, anxiety, stomach pains and huge emotional outbursts and asthma all disappeared. It became obvious that most of their problems were coming from the wrong diet and unhealthy gut. Maybe cooking everything from scratch is difficult, but not as difficult as constant doctors' visits and sick kids! Now we only go to the doctor for sports injuries, because my kids almost never get sick.

This diet and Dr Natasha Campbell-McBride saved my family, my marriage and my children. Thank you, thank you, thank you!

I only wish that everyone knew about a healthy gut before they got pregnant, so what my family went through could be avoided altogether.

A comment from Dr Natasha

Thank you, Eileen, for this story!

Like Eileen, many women now realize that there is NO WAY to have a healthy family without going back to the kitchen and cooking good quality fresh food for those you love! She has repeated twice that it is much easier to cook for your family fresh meals every day, than go though the misery of constant illness, medications and visits to hospitals.

There are many families such as this in the world, where children suffer from various health problems. A simple change in diet can bring so much happiness and normality into the family's life! Eileen has found the right information and had the strength and determination to save her family by changing the way they eat.

19

Kim Schuette

Certified GAPS Practitioner

Key words: bipolar disorder, recurrent ear infections, antibiotics

Getting at the Gut: A Solution for Treating Bipolar

The Merck Manual describes bipolar disorder as 'a condition in which periods of depression alternate with periods of mania or lesser degrees of excitement.' Historically known as manic-depressive disorder, this psychiatric condition is typically defined by the presence of abnormally elevated energy levels affecting mood and awareness, with or without states of depression. Manic states are often accompanied by psychotic symptoms such as delusions and hallucinations. Allopathic medicine's solution generally involves one or more pharmaceuticals for a lifetime and never offers a cure, but rather management of erratic behaviour via medications that often need to be changed from time to time. Quite commonly, those suffering from bipolar disorder are very bright, creative and loving individuals. Sadly, when brain chemistry goes out of balance, the person suffering with this disorder most often deals with chaos involving hallucinations, as well as extreme mania and rage.

Hippocrates, the father of modern medicine, once said 'All disease begins in the gut.' While not all individuals with gut dysbiosis experience psychological or psychiatric disease, I have yet (in 13 years of practice) to observe the absence of gut dysbiosis in those suffering from psychological or psychiatric challenges.

In September 2008, I had the privilege of meeting a very bright but troubled nine-year-old girl, whom I will call Mary. Mary had been diagnosed bipolar 11 months earlier by a psychiatrist. This conclusion came after years of deeply concerning behaviour. By the second grade, she was expelled from her private school due to her aggressive behaviour towards students and her teacher. This prompted her parents to make the decision to home-school her. Mary's mother quit her practice in the health field in order to give full-time attention to her daughter's daily needs. Prior to seeing the psychiatrist, Mary described in detail to her counsellor how she planned to kill herself some day. It was at this point that the counsellor and her parents realized that Mary needed serious help. Her parents' 'gut sense' was that pharmaceuticals would not offer the long-term solution they desired for their daughter. It was at this junction they were referred to my office. During my first meeting with the family, Mary was in a state of mild agitation with constant fidgeting and head shaking. She described the sensation of 'things crawling' in her head. Mary presented with a very red and expansive rash on her bottom, which had been longstanding.

Before focusing on Mary, I took a look first at her parents' health history and habits. I suspected that Mary might be a GAPS patient. GAPS is an acronym for Gut and Psychology Syndrome, based on the work of neurologist Natasha Campbell-McBride, M.D. This work finds that those individuals with psychiatric disorders, as well as depression, anxiety and ADD/ADHD, also have digestive problems. This is evidenced by many symptoms including (but not limited to) acne, allergies, asthma, constipation, diarrhoea, eczema and other skin rashes. Dr Campbell-McBride's findings echo the words of Hippocrates that 'all disease begins in the gut.' Given the GAPS research, and the fact that children inherit many gut and psychology issues from their parents, I examined her parents' histories.

Mary's mother had been a frequent user of the birth control pill and numerous rounds of antibiotics to address chronic bladder infections. She also had a history of vaginal yeast infections, which is common following the use of antibiotics. Antibiotics wipe out most bacteria, good and bad, leaving room on the mucosal lining of the gastrointestinal tract and the vaginal canal for opportunistic yeast to grow. Mary's mother also followed a typical American diet with an emphasis on low-fat foods, based on Dean Ornish's recommendations, prior to conception. Mary's father was addicted to sugar, Cokes and Oreos. He presented with chronic subcutaneous dermatitis, inflammation of the skin, most commonly seen as eczema. This condition is the result of imbalance of good flora in the gut. Both parents' diet had a history of strict adherence to the USDA's recommended food group of choice, grains. They both had used Acutane for the treatment of acne and appeared to suffer from the typical distressed liver function which generally follows Acutane usage.

The history of both parents gave me great insight into the weak links in Mary's development. Both parents suffered from gut dysbiosis. Both parents were unable to pass on good flora and strong immunity to their child due to their own weakened states (from diets composed primarily of processed foods, high in sugar and gluten, and their exposure to antibiotics and other pharmaceuticals).

I learned that Mary was conceived in the Sierra Mountains at a time when Lyme disease was widespread. Mary's mom was an avid hiker, as well as a veterinarian, making it likely that she had come in contact with the spirochete that causes Lyme disease. Research has shown that pathogens like the spirochete, Borrelia burgdorferi and its hitchhiking partners, Babesia, Ehrlichia, Bartonella, Mucoplasma and Anaplasma, can cross the placenta barrier and infect the developing child. A breached gut wall (due to abnormal gut flora) leaves a child or an adult vulnerable to pathogenic invaders and bacteria that are simply looking for a home. The gut wall barrier can become breached when there is an absence of life-giving, probiotic bacteria protecting the gut lining, and the presence of partially digested proteins (such as gluten), creating lesions in the gut lining. The result is impaired assimilation of nutrients along with inflammation. This is in part due to consuming highly refined grains not properly soaked and prepared. The lack of lacto-fermented foods is another contributing factor in developing a breached gut wall barrier.

Mary was born via C-section, therefore she would have missed out on the natural inoculation of friendly bacteria that should have been residing in the vaginal birth canal. However, due to mom's history of antibiotics, birth control pills and regular sugar consumption, she would have lacked sufficient beneficial bacteria to impart to Mary during delivery anyway. Mary was breastfed for 16 months. Nonetheless, she suffered from chronic constipation, beginning at five months of age. She was fed rice cereal with mineral oil per the advice of her paediatrician. Mineral oil, a petroleum-derived product, can be contaminated with cancer-causing PAH's (Polycyclic Aromatic Hydrocarbons), and is known to be immunosuppressive. (Petroleum-based products have been banned in the European Union since 2004.) Her paediatric gastroenterologist concluded 'nothing is wrong with Mary,' and confirmed the use of mineral oil.

After her first birthday, Mary had five years of chronic ear infections. Within this five-year period she was placed on 10 different antibiotics. At the age of four, her tonsils and adenoids were removed. The tonsils were so enlarged due to chronic infection that they were touching one another. As a result, Mary's snoring was so loud, it could be heard throughout the house.

Up until Mary entered kindergarten, her parents thought she was just very strong-willed and bright. Bright she was. Mary has an IQ of 140. But it was soon after she began the kindergarten that Mary's parents realized that her anger and behaviour were far from normal. Mary understood she was different from her peers. By first grade she was throwing chairs and other objects in the classroom at children, especially boys. She would threaten homicide to others. Despite many attempts by patient teachers trying to redirect her behaviour, Mary was uncontrollable. By the beginning of second grade, Mary was suspended. She would run down the hall at home flailing her arms and raging for two hours at a time. Often she crawled in between her mattress and box spring or buried herself under the bed for hours on end. Other times she would withdraw into herself and her books. (To date, at age 13, Mary has read over 2,200 books.) Many times Mary's eyes would 'flatline,' to use her father's words. She would become completely disconnected and unable to communicate. Often, after an hour and a half of head butting, biting, and raging, Mary would pass out and then wake up with words of apology.

As her parents saw Mary 'going dark,' they sought help from a local family therapist, who had a Ph.D. in education with an emphasis on gifted children. At the same time they began working with several neurological developmental specialists and, eventually, the psychiatrist who diagnosed Mary bipolar. All professionals agreed that Mary likely had a genius level IQ but, sadly, no long-term solutions for her disorder were offered. As her obstinate behaviour grew and threats of suicide increased, their therapist felt something immediate needed to be done. After four hours of meetings with the psychiatrist, the mood disorder diagnosis was given. The psychiatrist was reluctant to prescribe anti-psychotic drugs to such a young, smart child; Mary's parents agreed.

With full history in hand, we ran a comprehensive three-day stool test. Proper Lyme testing, which can be done through a specialty lab, is very costly and therefore the parents chose to forego the testing and begin addressing the diet and support for the gut. To best accomplish this, I recommended they use the Gut And Psychology Syndrome (GAPS) Diet as designed by neurologist Dr Natasha Campbell-McBride.

The GAPS Diet was a huge shift for this family of three whose diet had been primarily centred around refined carbohydrates with some low-fat dairy and meats. But in desperation, they made it a family affair. Within a few weeks, Mary's rash began disappearing. Within three months of beginning the GAPS Diet and our nutritional support, Mary's raging ended.

We limited her nutritional supplementation to Bio-Kult, minerals and Blue Ice Royal, a combination of X-factor butter oil and fermented cod liver oil. This combination was used often by Dr Weston A. Price in treating many different states of deficiency. Bio-Kult helped us to quickly populate Mary's gut with much needed beneficial bacteria as she adapted to eating lacto-fermented foods on a daily basis. The Blue Ice Royal, a rich source of vitamins A and D, and daily bone broth, supplying amino acids and minerals, provided all the nutrients needed to heal the gut lining. I also included homeopathic drainage remedies to assist her body in slowly eliminating toxins in the gut and the brain. Botanical tinctures were used to address infection in the body.

Mary and her parents agreed that the two biggest challenges presented by the GAPS Diet are the elimination of gluten and casein. The elimination of these is essential in healing the gut, which is almost always required in healing psychiatric conditions. One of the earliest works showing the effects of gluten on the brain was done by a psychiatrist F.Curtis Dohan, who noted that schizophrenic patients had fewer hospitalizations when bread become unavailable during World War II. This was seen throughout Canada, the United States, Finland,

Norway and Sweden. He found similar correlation in New Guinea, where schizophrenia was basically nonexistent in people on primitive diets until cultivated wheat products and beer made from barley (a gluten-containing grain) were introduced. At that point schizophrenia rates increased 65 fold.

One of the most extensive clinical trials of our time regarding food and behaviour took place in Denmark. Fifty-five autistic children were placed on a gluten and casein-free diet. Tremendous improvement in behaviour was seen in these children. Dr Dohan and his colleagues at the Veterans Administration Hospital in Philadelphia saw similar results in schizophrenic patients in the mid-sixties after putting patients on a gluten-free diet for four weeks. There was a reduced number of auditory hallucinations, delusion and less social detachment. Once gluten was reintroduced, the disturbing behaviours returned. Obviously not everyone who is gluten or casein sensitive exhibits the extreme symptoms of autism or schizophrenia. But other health issues may ensue when the gut wall lining has been breached. Allergies, acne, eczema, and gastrointestinal complaints are just a few of the symptoms that can point to gut dysbiosis. I have found the GAPS Programme to be the body's best support for healing. Prior to using the GAPS Diet in 2005, I saw the Specific Carbohydrate Diet assist many to a certain degree of wellness. The GAPS Diet, however, because of its emphasis on nutrient-dense, gut-healing foods, can bring complete healing to those with gut disorders.

Several months after I began working with Mary, we retested her stool to find that the high levels of previously detected MRSA (methyl-resistant staphylococcus aureus) had left her body. Over the next nine months her behaviour gradually normalized. Exactly a year from beginning the GAPS Diet, Mary and her parents attended a family reunion where family members were shocked at Mary's transformation!

Today, Mary is a vivacious, happy, normal 13-year-old, still reading books and bringing laughter to those around her. Her kind and loving spirit touches all who are blessed to know her. Mary is fortunate to have parents dedicated to her healing!

Today, modern cultures are seeing soaring rates of ADD/ADHD, allergies, autism and psychiatric disorders in the very young, as refined carbohydrates, particularly modified gluten products produced in 60 minutes or less, and pasteurized, denatured dairy products continue to dominate diets. More and more research points to the wisdom of Hippocrates that 'all disease begins in the gut.' Hippocrates also offered this insight: *'I know, too, that the body is affected differently by bread according to the manner in which it is prepared. It differs according as it is made from pure flour or meal with bran, whether it is prepared from winnowed or unwinnowed wheat, whether it is mixed with much water or little, whether well mixed or poorly mixed, over-baked or under-baked, and countless other points besides. The same is true of the preparation of barley meal. The influence of each process is considerable and each has a totally different effect from another. How can anyone who has not considered such matters and come to understand them possibly know anything of the diseases that afflict mankind? Each one of the substances of a man's diet acts upon his body and changes it in some way and upon these changes his whole life depends.'*

This truth is never more evident than today. We are bearing the consequences of departure from traditional food preparations in exchange for modern technology and so?called convenience. The fall-out lies in the minds and guts of our young! The good news is that our bodies are capable of self?healing. As we return to the wisdom of our ancient forefathers and foremothers, we can help our children to recapture their potential for wellness.

A comment from Dr Natasha

I am so proud of my Certified GAPS Practitioners! Thank you, Kim, for this wonderful story and for your work! Yes, psychiatric conditions are born in the gut, all of them (I have no doubt)! The treatment has to focus on healing the gut and re-establishing healthy gut flora. What kind of life and what kind of a future did Mary have with her bipolar disorder?... A simple change in diet has given this child a normal and happy life, and a very bright future! Thank you for quoting Hippocrates, Kim; he is absolutely right – food is extremely powerful, probably the most powerful influence on human health (and the most underestimated).

20

Kathleen Mills

Key words: adopted child, childhood schizophrenia / autism, addiction to sugar

'To laugh often and much; to win the respect of intelligent people and the affection of children; to earn the appreciation of honest critics and to endure the betrayal of false friends. To appreciate beauty; to find the best in others; to leave the world a bit better whether by a healthy child, a garden patch, or a redeemed social condition; to know that even one life has breathed easier because you have lived. This is to have succeeded.' – *Ralph Waldo Emerson*

My son, Matthew's, 12th birthday was yesterday. He calmly blew out his birthday candle, and proudly announced, 'See, Mom! I'm growing into a man.' Not that many years ago, he would have shrieked, terrorized by the candle's flame, or the ripping-sound of birthday gift wrap, torn free from his presents. I could never have imagined, 11 years ago, the loving, gentle-natured, articulate boy he has become.

We met our son the first time the day we adopted him. He was 11 months old, but developmentally he was the equivalent of a two-month-old. I'd like to have held him in my arms, but he'd have nothing to do with us, his shoulders locked into a stiff, rigid position, making him impossible to hold.

During the four-hour paper-signing process, Matthew screamed at the top of his lungs, head-butting anyone who offered comfort. His poor little face – swollen and red from the effort – bore no resemblance to the sweet-faced baby in the photos sent to us by the adoption agency. We explained away his behaviour: he was shy, we were strangers, and he was in an unfamiliar environment. As the hours wore on, the screams more insistent, my husband and I exchanged raised eyebrows communicating, "What are we getting ourselves into?"

Our despair didn't go unnoticed by the agency director who suggested we retreat into her office for a cup of tea while she "reviewed Matthew's file, just one last time". We sipped, while she flipped through Matthew's file. "Here's a recent doctor's evaluation – written two weeks ago – that I don't think you've seen", she remarked, and then read, "...given proper structure, care, feeding, consistent parenting and love, developmental delays will diminish." The adoption agency director concluded, "I'm not sure what's wrong with Matthew. And to be honest, I think he's high-risk. I'm sure you'll find a good doctor who can provide you with more information."

Houseplants came with better instructions!

With hearts full of hope, and a refilled diaper-bag that included a fresh tube of Nystatin for Matthew's 'pervasive fungus issues', we flew home with our son. For the next four years, I researched, arranged appointments with 'professionals' and 'experts', often waiting anywhere from 12 weeks to 12 months for our appointments. The more specialized the doctor or evaluator, the longer we had to wait.

I'd left the corporate world behind, but used my management skills to form a medical 'team', asking our developmental paediatrician to be the 'lead'. For the first round of meetings, everyone agreed that results from EEG, MRI and BEAM (brain electrical activity mapping), as well as some basic blood work, were needed to eliminate or confirm the existence of medical conditions – brain tumours, seizures, and Fragile-X – which might explain some of Matthew's symptoms and behaviours.

- Scented products triggered immediate black circles underneath his eyes;
- Within 20 minutes of eating, he'd scream and clutch his arms and legs, complaining of sharp pains;
- Large blisters covered his inner thighs immediately following bowel movements;

- Unable to discern between hot and cold water or weather, he insisted on wearing winter clothes in scorching summer heat, and summer clothes in below-zero temperatures;
- Lacked ability to generalize (screamed when placed into a car seat, then screamed when taken out of a car seat);
- School 'experts' reported odd behaviours – trance-like state, conversing with 'make-believe friends';
- Increased nightmares and night-frights;
- Limited vocabulary, repetitive sounds and perseveration (repetition, echoing) replaced meaningful communication until age four;
- Developed permanent purple discoloration on forehead from head-banging on walls, floors, chair legs and his mattress;
- Self-mutilation – ripped chunks of flesh from his face during periods of silence;
- Sudden noises sent him running face-first into brick walls or glass doors;
- Auditory and visual hallucinations of footsteps, voices and seeing people: in our home who 'talked' to him, giving him instructions;
- Bowel movement colours ranged from pure white, purple, orange, green, gold and near-black, but seldom brown; textures varied from liquid to dry sawdust.

During a psychiatric evaluation, he refused to sit quietly near the evaluator, but instead bolted under the conference table, leaped out the opposite side, making a mad dash toward the full-length third-floor glass window. We intercepted him a split-second before he would have made full-body contact with the glass. Later, he said his intent was to 'fly into the sky'.

An acquaintance, a retired psychiatrist, commented, 'There is a reason the U.S. Navy codes autism as schizophrenia.' Another well-intentioned friend suggested exorcism as a 'cure'.

An impending diagnosis of early-onset childhood-schizophrenia, at the tender age of four, received the attention and interest of world-renowned autism researchers from Cambridge and Harvard, Massachusetts. We accepted their invitation to meet at their next available opening – 11 months away.

A Pattern Emerges

During the interim, our new doctors asked me to present them with compiled notes and journal entries I'd created over the years, which described my son's hallucinations, sleep patterns, food preferences, and complaints of physical pain. On a whim, I created a timeline detailing repetitive behaviours I'd noticed. A pattern emerged: every six weeks Matthew's behaviour degenerated, beginning with bright-gold bowel movements (which I realized marked the beginning of a downward spiral) followed by markedly increased aggression, self-limiting intake of foods, complaints of arm and head-pain (which our son described 'like ants crawling through his brain'). Sleep patterns were disrupted with increased head-banging, severe night-frights, as well as auditory and visual hallucinations.

Around the third week, I noted bowel movements were like sawdust, 'stuff of nightmares', as if he were a teddy-bear losing his stuffing. Over the next few weeks, his body rebounded – behaviour calmed down, appetite increased, good sleep patterns returned as did his self-control, both at home and school. Near the end of the sixth week, his bowel movements also improved, nearing the standard of 'normal' coloration, albeit never solid.

It was the third week – the middle of the cycle – that was the most difficult for our entire family, especially during meal times. Even though high-carb food had been banned, he still tried to throw his weight around, insisting we restore crackers, pasta, extruded cereal and grocery-store bread. His aggressive tactics destroyed plates and bowls of food, which he swept to the floor. Worse, he was skilled in using projectile vomiting against family members and their dinners. He also 'pocketed' food in his cheeks to the point they looked ready to burst – less destructive to our appetites – but nonetheless nerve wracking, as we were concerned that he would choke.

Ever-creative, a sure sign of an intelligent mind, Matthew's dinner-time tactics to acquire sugar-loaded food became more aggressive. One evening, when I approached the dinner table, carrying bowls of food, he suddenly leaped up, stood on his chair, and delivered a full-scale scream into my left ear. Its force pitched me forward, sending bowls flying from my hands. I bent low over the table, my hands placed squarely on the table surface trying to regain my balance. Out of the corner of my eye, I saw Matthew inhale, readying himself to delivery another sonic blast. Instinctively, I grabbed a large pickled cucumber from a serving plate, and inserted it into his cavernous mouth. Silence!.. My spirit felt crushed and I immediately repented, convinced I'd just slipped across the line into child abuse. Through tears, I watched as Matthew's contorted, rage-bloated face relaxed. He grabbed the pickle, inspected it, and took a huge bite. His face softened, his smile angelic – this was the face of a stranger, a sweet child previously unknown to us. I sat down at the table with my exhausted family, our dinners forgotten, as we watched Matthew cherishing each and every bite of the traditional half-sour cucumber. He turned to me, and asked for more, even using the word, "Please"!

Fermented Foods Were Key!

Properly-fermented foods, like the half-sour cucumber, turned out to be the missing key! When Matthew developed a taste for the pickled cukes, he became excited to try other fermented foods – cultured butter, yogurt, sauerkraut, kraut juice, pickled carrots - delivering important probiotic bacteria and living enzymes. (A few years later, I discovered that food scientists classify properly fermented vegetables as 'bitter', which physically switches the tongue's sweet receptors off, so the tongue is more receptive to sour and bitter tastes. That was the switch we needed to break Matthew's sugar addiction, which had been created by his birth grandmother who gave him sugar water instead of whole foods.)

We saw real changes. His bowel movements became solid for the first time in five years of his life. He was calmer, more focused. Two weeks into the diet, he announced, 'I'm going to bed early,' and, for the first time, slept through the night. Not long after Matthew's marked improvement, the school district's assistant director of special needs phoned and accused us of placing our son on medication without informing them. I met with her and the entire educational team, explaining we'd 'put Matthew on food, not drugs'. Matthew's occupational and speech therapists, classroom teacher, one-on-one aid, behaviourist, psychologist, and school nurse listened intently as we explained the Weston A. Price Foundation's dietary guidelines we'd followed for the past 30 days. Most everyone, with the exception of the school district representative, applauded our efforts. Matthew's teacher said, "..His behaviour changes, within such a short time, are nothing short of a miracle". The school nurse, who allowed our son to use her private bathroom, added she was, "... amazed that his stools are hard! I had never seen a kid with such awful diarrhoea, so whatever you are doing, keep doing it!"

The more our son progressed and the more his troubling behaviours diminished, the more we understood that nutrient-dense properly-prepared food was crucial to his well-being. The challenge became that not everyone on Matthew's school 'team' wanted to go along with what some considered 'too-restrictive' a diet. One occupational therapist complained, "Without candy or gum, I can't get him to obey!"

Nutrition Confirmed

We removed our son from public school, choosing home-schooling, and continued to focus on nutrition as healing. At the end of our 11-month wait, we met with our new team of Cambridge and Harvard doctors that included Dr Martha Herbert, a world-renowned expert in autism. When we settled into comfortable chairs, seated in front of her desk, she sat back, folded her hands and said, "tell me everything".

Dr Herbert listened without interrupting. She confirmed several of my ideas about the link between nutrition and Matthew's symptoms, which others had mocked as fantastical notions. 45 minutes later, I had said everything I'd come to say, everything that I needed someone with her knowledge to hear – for verification, correction, or erudition.

'Do you know what you are?' she asked, after a few moments of silence. My mind fired off a wide range of responses – tired, inquisitive, weary, tenacious – but before I answered, she continued. "Do you know, you're not alone? You have peers, a large team of researchers just like you. I have a name for all of you – Poopologists. It's not a fancy name. But it is a noble endeavour, and one for which I have the deepest, most profound respect and admiration. You are practising important science. I'm just here to back you up, to attempt to validate, find the science to explain what you already know.'

'If you think of it as a brain disorder that's a miswiring from birth, then what the parents are doing is utterly insane or incongruous. But if you think of the brain as being affected by the whole body, then when you affect the body, you can affect the brain. And that's the rationale of what parents are doing. The parents are doing, in my view, systems biology. I think that parents have beat medicine to systems biology.' – *Dr Martha Herbert.*

Dr Herbert concluded her evaluation, finding no symptoms of early-onset childhood schizophrenia, which had existed prior to the change in Matthew's diet. She explained the results of comprehensive stool and blood-panels as being "Abnormally normal!" – wonderful news! Dr Herbert credited Matthew's diet and told us to "not change a thing". She also had a theory that Matthew's six-week cycles were either fungus or bacteria-driven; that when he emptied himself with severe bouts of diarrhoea, he cleaned the 'critters' out, but that when they built up again in his intestines, the cycle began all over again. As we continued giving a wide range of properly created anaerobic-fermented foods, being careful to protect the food from oxygen (so as not to develop oxygen-rich yeasts or mould that would irritate his system), the six-week cycles diminished, fully extinguished by his seventh birthday.

Dr Natasha's *Gut and Psychology Syndrome* is a valuable resource, a tool I wish I'd had when we were first beginning to unravel the mystery of our son's 'condition'. I urge everyone I talk to about food and health-related topics to read GAPS. If ever there was a wise maintenance manual for the proper care and feeding of the human digestive, nervous and brain system, GAPS is it!

A comment from Dr Natasha

Thank you, Kathleen! What a story! It is full of insight and helpful information for other parents who have to deal with similar problems in their children. Recent research shows that our gut flora constitutes 90% of all cells and genetic material in the human body. If these 90% of us are dominated by pathogens nothing in the body can function normally. Matthew's situation is a clear demonstration of that! Bringing gut flora to normality spells a difference between a 'nightmare child' and a sweet healthy little boy – a joy to bring up.

Motivated by their son's needs, Kathleen Mills and her husband Mark created the popular Pickl-It system (an optimal anaerobic fermentation system), that creates consistent, clean-quality, probiotic-rich, beneficial fermented foods – an essential part of the GAPS diet. I highly recommend it, particularly for those who are trying fermentation for the first time.

21

Gabriela Mikova

Key words: autism, depression, allergies, eczema, asthma, poor immunity, digestive disorders, mental illness, migraines, malnourishment

My name is Gabriela. I am 34 years old. English is my foreign language but I will do my best to tell my story.

Since I was a little girl I have had hallucinations. It was hard to know sometimes what reality was and what was my imagination. As a child I had bad eczema and outdoor allergies. I remember missing a lot of school because of constant colds, flu and sickness. I had anxiety issues, hives and panic attacks. I was toe-walking all my childhood. Transitions were hard for me. I was running away from school from first to third grade. I feared other children. I could not fit in a classroom. It was hard to have friends. I wondered what was I doing in this world? I so wanted to have friends, but kids called me weird, because I could not understand right away or exactly what they meant or wanted from me.

When my menstruations started I was bleeding too heavily and had lots of cramps, I started having migraines, stomach upsets and a lot of abdominal pain. From 15 I was put on a contraceptive pill; still I bled 5–9 times per month. They gave me hormonal injections.

Around the age of 16–17 I developed depression. I was sad all the time, so much sadness in this world! My parents were loving and caring people, and I could not describe where this sadness was coming from. I took relationships very seriously. I thought that when I got a boyfriend, it would be forever. When a break-off came I could not let it go. Sometimes I rocked myself to calm down and I was crying, crying and crying. Once I wrote my sadness on a piece of paper and my father found it in my bed. He got so sad, he could not understand why I was so unhappy, and he blamed himself.

I heard voices in my head all the time. Sometimes the voices told me to do bad things. I fought to ignore them. At the age of 17 I was seriously underweight (38 kilograms) and was losing weight, and I was so sad and depressed. Sometimes I would lose consciousness. I suffered with constant joint pain and yeast infections. I was also anaemic. I had a lot of headaches.

Around 20 I wanted to end my life a couple of times. I could not find a good job, I was always looking to do something that would have purpose and meaning. In 2001 I moved to the USA with my boyfriend. There things got even worse. I was feeling that I did not have my own life under control, like there was something controlling my life, as if somebody put mysterious fog around me and I could not see through. The joint pains got a lot worse, and so did allergies and migraines. My mental symptoms got worse, but I was afraid to talk to anyone about it.

In 2006 I got pregnant. I was vomiting from the beginning to the end of the pregnancy. On 16 March 2007 I gave birth to my son Matthew after a long and difficult labour. He appeared to be healthy, weighed 7 lb 4 oz and was 21 inches long. But everything I thought to be beautiful turned into a nightmare. I suffered from postnatal depression and Matthew was screaming non-stop. Without any help I did not know how we could make it. After his first vaccinations Matthew developed terrible eczema all over his body. He was crying extra hard and even longer, arching his back. He had a nappy rash and started to get constipated, despite being breastfed. Around 18 months of age he developed a bad cough and was diagnosed with asthma. I also noticed that he was not doing what other children started to do: imaginative play, more talking. Matt was always on the go, crying, irritated by everything.

I got pregnant again. Around this time Matthew limited his food to starch and dairy only. He was constantly crying 5–6 hours at night. I used to rock him for an hour, he would sleep for 20 minutes and then start crying again. His asthma worsened, the doctor gave us pneumacord and nebulizers (steroids). These things only made him worse. We were living a nightmare! I had more and more concerns and nobody had answers. Matthew continued to be sick. At the age of three he was very constipated having a bowel movement once every three-four-five days. He became a very finicky eater.

After recommended vaccinations at the age of three and a flu shot we had pest control at our home (because of an insect problem), and something else started to happen to our son. He became very distant, very pale and his speech started disappearing. He acted as if confused. He could not understand what we were saying to him. He was running in small circles and started having giggling episodes. We were losing him. His constipation worsened – one stool every six to eight days, his bottom was hurting and he bled when passing stool. We tried vitamin C, magnesium, dry plums – nothing worked. I had my own problems too which did not help the situation. My mood was swinging from a raging anger to melancholy.

My breaking point was when Matt did not have a bowel movement for nine days. I called one lady who owns a natural food shop in NJ. After a couple of hours talking she handed me your book, Dr Natasha, *Gut And Psychology Syndrome*, and said that I should follow the book as closely as possible!

That was our turning point. I read the first few pages of your book and cried, cried and cried. I started to keep a diary of what I and Matthew ate. I started to exclude gluten. First we went off grains, and my son started to sleep through the night. WOW, that was huge! Then I took Matthew off all the steroids. Than I took milk protein out: WOW, he stopped crying and became less confused! I started to do everything according to your book. I was worried at the beginning that we would starve because I was a terrible cook.

My daughter Anna was born in June 2009. I breastfed her, yet by four months she got terribly constipated. After the usual vaccinations at seven months she barely moved, stopped babbling and stopped looking around. I put her on GAPS at the age of eight months. At that point I decided to refuse any further vaccinations for my children. I felt that they have done enough damage to them already!

We have been on the GAPS Programme since Matt's third birthday. Everybody thought I was crazy, especially my husband. But by the third week of being truly gluten-free I stopped hearing voices, and the angry raging stopped. My eczema and joint pains lessened, and my headaches stopped. I am not confused anymore: I can drive anywhere and find my way home. I am more confident than I ever was. The oversensitive crying stopped. No more heavy dreams and nightmares!

I just wish I had found this knowledge before, especially for my children!

When I gave birth to my daughter Anna in 2009, the second day doctors vaccinated me. They just came in and gave me a shot without any explanation. Since then I was very sick to the point of being diagnosed with Crohn's disease, anaphylactic allergy and rheumatism. Doctors had no idea what was wrong with me. Today I am as good as new thanks to the GAPS Diet, juicing, raw foods, probiotics, fermented food and supplements. I found books by Norman W. Walker also very helpful.

We tried DAN with a lot of expense for Matthew (we could not afford to do it for both children!). But we have something better now: we have your book, Dr Natasha! I do believe that with GAPS Protocol you can help anybody, not only those who have money. Home cooking is time-consuming indeed, but so healthy and worth it, especially if you have small children!

By writing this letter I have an opportunity to be heard. GAPS works, people! GAPS saved my life! It helped me to get my health back so now I am in charge of my life and can take care of the ones I love! Especially if my loved ones have serious problems, such as autism.

Today my son is four years and six months. He is highly social, loves children, smiles and is a happy child. He says three to four word sentences. We teach him two languages at the same time, so it is a lot, but he is getting there. He asks: Mommy, what is next? He is due to start ABA programme soon, and I know he'll be just fine, he is really ready to learn and he is interested in learning. I had my doubts on the way, but I am so glad I stayed the path!

Anna started talking at two, her muscle tone improved and she walks well now; she is not distant anymore. At 18 months she appeared to be deaf; now she responds just fine, only her speech is a bit delayed. But, she does not meet criteria for autism anymore!

We have a lot of work ahead of us, but we will get there! Last year I went to the Weston A. Price Foundation conference in PA. I could not miss the opportunity to see Dr Natasha's presentation! I told my husband: it is either the conference or I'll keep phoning England! Conference was a cheaper option! I got the revised edition of the book with your signature. It was a pleasure to meet you Doctor, in person!

Because of what happened to my family, I am now considering getting an education in nutrition. People should realize that IT IS NOT OK TO EAT PROCESSED FOOD and that it is NECESSARY TO GET OUR BUTTS BACK TO THE KITCHEN! Because we are not only what we eat, we are mostly what we can digest!

Forgive me, I am not too good at writing, but I sincerely hope that my letter can encourage other people, parents not to give up! If I could do it, they can do it too! I will be happy to offer any support I can to those who struggle the way I did. They can contact me at konteska0nine@gmail.com . This is how much I believe in and trust in your work, Dr Natasha! I sincerely hope that you can save as many lives as possible, because there is nothing more beautiful than a smile on somebody's face!

A comment from Dr Natasha

What a humbling story! Thank you, Gabriela! This story shows again that there are no hopeless situations. Any person, no matter how ill, can regain their health and get their life back!

I will be delighted to train you as a GAPS Practitioner when you are ready, Gabriela. People like you make the best practitioners because you have lived the programme; you have precious experience, which cannot be replaced by anything else in the world! And you have a big heart! Thank you!

22

J.F.

Key words: mental illness, hyperactivity, fussy eating, sugar addiction, sleeping problems, allergies, overuse of antibiotics, headaches, poor immunity, yeast infection, PMS

My daughter is recovering from a mental illness! I want to shout it from the rooftops! I should correct myself; she's recovering from a probable diagnosis of mental illness, as the reader will soon see.

Alex had a few symptoms in her early years; most notably hyperactivity (improved when corn syrup was eliminated) and poor dietary and sleep habits. During her early school years she would demand candy at every opportunity; her eyes hard and glittery, her body tensed for battle. I learned to avoid grocery shopping with her and candy was limited to holidays. She gave up eating meat at age 10. At age 11 she had a pneumonia, which was difficult to treat, that set off a wave of respiratory illnesses, some legitimate, some I now believe were an allergic reaction to powdered corn stirred up in the chicken coop.

Between the ages of 12 and 14 her behavioural symptoms spiralled out of control, worsening each year. We were in a vicious cycle: often she would have lower respiratory-like symptoms and feel ill. She would refuse to attend school until she was better, often missing more than a week. The public school administration required a doctor's note for students missing five or more days, which would always result in a prescription for preventative antibiotics. I was very concerned by the number of times Alex was put on antibiotics, but she needed to return to school and there was always that anxiety of a developing bronchitis or pneumonia.

One October day near Halloween we reached a crisis. She was 14 and had recently started her freshman year of high school. She'd had yet another lower respiratory-like illness treated with antibiotics. Every school day started the same. A dark blanket covered her windows to block out light. I'd enter her room at 6a.m. to wake her. She'd feign sleep or she'd argue, scream and try to kick me or throw things. Her siblings complained their Halloween candy was missing and I found wrappers all over the house and candy stashed in Alex's drawer. One missed week of school turned into two, then three, then six. When awake, she'd follow me around the house continually demanding to know why I wouldn't allow a puppy or other obsessions. Her confrontational behaviour was verbally aggressive and sometimes turned physical. Her younger brother had to be kept in separate rooms as her behaviour toward him was intolerable.

I argued with school officials to keep my daughter in school without involving the law. To protect my daughter's privacy, I did not fully disclose our situation. Perhaps that was a mistake. Alex could not fall asleep until three in the morning and she would not awaken until mid-afternoon. Her hair was tangled and dirty, her room smelled horrible. If I wasn't home when she was awake she would bake desserts to satisfy her intense cravings for sugar.

Her symptoms appearing over that three-year time period were:

- Extreme anger, bullying and aggression, both physical and verbal, usually directed at her younger brother;
- Very confrontational and argumentative;
- Paranoid and beginning to hallucinate;
- Repetitive behaviours such as jerking her head to one side and touching a certain spot on the wall;
- Frequent spitting;
- Extreme menstrual pain;
- Sensitive to light, noise, smells and temperature;
- Refused to cooperate, leave her room or attend school;
- Occasional unexplained vaginal yeast infections;
- Extreme fatigue and unwillingness to participate in anything;
- Often complained of dizziness, gas pains in her tummy, and vomiting;
- Complained of headaches, sore throats and lower respiratory symptoms*;

- Often had a red rashy ring around her mouth*;
- Insomnia and poor sleeping patterns;
- Foggy headed, confused and a poor ability to focus: math and languages were a particular problem at school;
- Obsessed about things and would go on about them for days;
- Symptoms worsened following a sugar binge, improved following a dose of probiotics or an all-vegetable meal.

* These symptoms disappeared when powdered corn and pineapple were eliminated.

I provided her paediatrician with a full list of her symptoms. I also supplied a two-week food-mood journal, documenting Alex's behaviour in relation to her eating patterns. Her doctor said she didn't see a pattern. Given Alex's food cravings and occasional rash I felt there was an allergy. The doctor handed me a page listing over 100 different environmental and food allergens. I could select whatever individual tests I wanted. They were expensive. I did not know what to choose and we were without health care at that time.

Did I mention my degree in microbiology? I knew the risk of Candidiasis when repeated use of antibiotics has shifted the balance of microflora in the gut. I suggested this as a possibility to Alex's paediatrician and that was dismissed as unlikely as her yeast infections were infrequent and she did not have oral thrush. A full psychiatric evaluation was recommended. At that point we transferred Alex to an online high school, and I was introduced to the incredible GAPS Diet.

I need to interrupt myself at this point to give the reader more background. My sister was diagnosed in her early 20s with schizophrenia affective disorder. She had similar eating and behavioural patterns with digestive issues. Her anger and aggression were usually directed towards me. She was in and out of mental institutions; she would walk the streets for hours and talk to trees. Sometimes she would stop taking her medications and then she became suicidal. I was willing to try ANYTHING to keep my daughter from that horrible life! Looking at my sister and parents today they are a family in crisis and need the GAPS Diet immediately, but they won't listen. My father has suffered from mood swings, poor focus, high blood pressure and ulcerative colitis for decades and may now need surgery for the colitis; my Mom has multiple sclerosis, a low level of chronic yeast infections and was recently diagnosed with diabetes; my sister's mental illness is under some degree of control with the combination of medications she's on now. An unfortunate side effect of the meds is tremendous weight gain, and she has acid reflux and irritable bowel syndrome.

Given the multi-generational family history of gut dysbiosis, the reader may wonder what my health is like. As a child I was very foggy-headed and emotional. I had some minor repetitive behaviours and suffered frequent migraines and abdominal discomfort in my teen years. My daughter's hyperactivity and sugar cravings when young led me to research nutrition and strive for a mostly whole food, organic diet. Today I feel fine. I've never liked bitter or sweet foods and I instinctively shun foods that are wrong for my body.

Alex's symptoms and my family's health history fell into place when I read the GAPS book. It was very difficult to convince a 14-year-old to try this diet, but as far as I was concerned it was not optional. If she refused I was prepared to have her confined to the house with nothing available to eat that was not GAPS legal. Fortunately, she consented to give it a try. I saw positive changes within two weeks. If she was tempted to cheat she'd experience gas pains, yeast infections and behavioural changes; that feedback keeps her on track.

Commitment to the GAPS Diet hasn't been easy; it must be given priority. In the early days Alex had chronic fatigue and was constantly hungry as she still refused to eat meat. I spent the majority of my day cooking, cleaning and caring for her. I introduced honey and fruit much too early, and we paid for it with several more weeks of health and behavioural issues. There were times when I was utterly exhausted and I have to admit it was tempting to give up, but I knew medications weren't the answer.

Alex has been on the GAPS Diet a year now and she's like a completely different child. She's happy, engaged and cooperative (for a teenager), and I have to say the sweetest moments are when she and her brother have a real conversation or collaborate on a project. Today her only symptoms are a somewhat irregular sleep pattern and one minor repetitive behaviour. We recently celebrated her 16th birthday with honey-sweetened home-made ice cream. She's worked hard and I'm very proud of her.

Permit me to include one more story. A few days ago in a park, while working on this piece, two overweight teenage girls sat at a nearby table. One said she was eating her favourite lunch of Doritos and Sprite. Later at our home that same evening, lentil soup was on the menu. My girls were voluntarily chopping vegetables while my husband washed dishes and our son entertained the new puppy. I stood by, marvelling at the scene.

Thank you, Dr Natasha, for sharing your wonderful work; it has given us back our child!

J.F. New Hampshire, USA

A comment from Dr Natasha

Thank you for this wonderful story! It is sad to say that this story is very typical: uncountable numbers of children and teenagers in our modern world suffer from sugar addiction and mental problems. The mental problems can be as mild as some mental fog and inability to concentrate (and hence underachieving at school), or full-blown mood swings, aggressive and unreasonable behaviour, obsessions, depression, psychosis and suicide.

J.F. is absolutely right: medication is not the answer! We have to deal with the root cause of the problem: the child's gut flora and diet. I am sure that now Alex has a good prospect of leading a healthy, normal and successful life!

23

M.C.

Key words: OCD (Obsessive Compulsive Disorder), PANDAS (Paediatric Autoimmune Neuropsychiatric Disorder Associated with Streptococcal infection), large doses of probiotics

At age 12, my daughter became very ill. She manifested with severe OCD. She was delusional and her behaviour bizarre. She totally withdrew from all social situations. It was utterly heartbreaking for her, her father, and me. As a baby, my daughter got lots of antibiotics from my milk when I was treated for a serious infection. We suspected that she might have PANDAS – Paediatric Autoimmune Neuropsychiatric Disorders Associated with Streptococcal infection. Our physician at the time was extremely unhelpful, so we treated her ourselves with strong doses of broad spectrum probiotics, based on our knowledge that beneficial microbes can bring down the pathogenic ones. She immediately and steadily improved. We also put her on fermented cod liver oil in hefty quantities and a nutrient-dense diet.

A year and a half later, although much improved, she still had residual intrusive thoughts. A new physician, who was affiliated through the Weston Price Foundation, had heard of your work and advised me that 'intrusive thoughts were related to gut flora.' I would have been astonished except for my familiarity with PANDAS and the idea that an infectious agent could cause neuro-psychiatric symptoms. A month after that, yet another Weston Price fan told me the same, while urging me to get Dr Campbell-McBride's book. As a result, I upped my daughter's probiotics considerably to very large doses. From that very moment on, she never had another intrusive thought. Not a single one. They completely and definitively subsided.

We chose, a year later, to begin the GAPS Diet. This latter effort has resulted in her tummy problems improving, as well as her stamina and strength. (She seems notably stronger than some of her peers.) She has gained weight; she used to be rail-thin; she is absorbing her foods now. There are some concerns that we still have with regard to focusing issues and mild hyperactivity, which we hope will resolve on the GAPS. She does spend her days at a school with wireless networking surrounding her, which I believe does not help issues one bit.

What I wish to share is that she benefited even before we started the GAPS Diet simply by the aggressive addition of the probiotics (introduced carefully and gradually), good quality probiotics and in healthy doses. I think this is important, because some mothers may feel so overwhelmed coping with their children's illnesses that they cannot even conceive of beginning with the diet. The probiotics enabled us to do something proactive immediately, which alleviated a sense of helplessness on our part. And because they also helped improve our daughter's serious symptoms, this greatly lifted some of the stress for our family, enabling us to consider a more long-term protocol. Let's face it: GAPS is a huge and challenging adjustment, but clearly well worth it.

A comment from Dr Natasha

Thank you for this story! M.C. made a very valuable point for parents who, for various reasons, cannot change their child's diet immediately. There are good supplements you can use, and therapeutic-strength probiotics are one of the first to consider. It is important to start from a small dose and build it up gradually to control the die-off reaction. Many people accomplished a lot of healing by simply taking good quality probiotics and other supplements.

24

Anne

Key words: PANDAS, ADHD, Oppositional Defiant Disorder, autism, extreme emotional instability, Chronic Fatigue Syndrome, lupus, eczema, digestive problems, depression, failure to thrive, asthma, hay fever, vaccine damage, food intolerances, hair loss

Our pre-GAPS life was getting harder. Our three and a half-year old Harriet had ADHD, I believed (the paediatrician wouldn't diagnose kids under the age of seven). Her behaviour at this time included daily screaming at the top of her lungs for hours, having berserk 'meltdown' episodes of hitting, kicking, screaming and repeatedly throwing her whole body against the wall. Harriet was constantly jumping and running, and seemed unable to stand or sit still or do any activity requiring concentration for long. She was an impulsive, reckless child that was quickly drawn to anything dangerous around. She would jump from a height and land on her knees repeatedly until restrained. Harriet also had Oppositional Defiant Disorder (which was diagnosed). She would scream loudly in response to any and every request put to her; "no way, I'm never going to do what you ask!" She also seemed to have PANDAS (a psychiatric condition triggered by *streptococcus* bacteria). Whenever she had a sore 'strep throat' (which was most of the time) she would start screaming uncontrollably and going wilder than usual, becoming violent and throwing herself around the room. This would sometimes last all day. She also had debilitating tummy aches daily, eczema, food intolerances and walked only on her tiptoes. A naturally extroverted child, she would scream at her friends to go home, and then remain in her room whilst we had visitors.

We tried a low-allergy, completely additive-free diet. Harriet had shown strong initial improvement, but after one year of eating this way many of her behaviours were worsening. In hindsight I understand why: the diet was excessively high in refined carbohydrates and potatoes while most detoxifying foods were avoided. Managing her care was often impossible, as she was too violent to enable us to bathe her or change her nappy. We could not take her out, not even to the playground opposite our house, as there was inevitably going to be screaming and kicking to such a degree that getting her home was fraught with difficulty.

As for me I began to realize that I had many signs of autism, and while these were perhaps not overt they had caused me to feel socially inept most of my adult life. I also suffered from extreme emotional over-reactions to very minor incidents. The feelings of rage and emotional pain were so intense; I would feel swamped and utterly overtaken by them. At these times I was unable to access any logical reasoning to mitigate my emotions. This is similar to what I've read about PANDAS, so perhaps I had my own psychiatric condition going on. It was very hard to control myself when my emotions were so out of control. I was afraid I was going to become violent. I had been on the same low-allergy diet as Harriet for a year and had experienced cravings for alcohol that were becoming more frequent and almost uncontrollable, although I had been abstinent for two years. I believe that this was due to my body manufacturing alcohol from all the refined carbohydrates in my diet. I also had a history of diarrhoea for 15 years, and constipation/diarrhoea for five months (since the birth of my son), Chronic Fatigue Syndrome, asthma, hay fever, food intolerances and hair loss.

My husband, Bernard, had been on the low-allergy and additive-free diet with us for a year also. His depression had deepened over that period to the point where he could only work part-time. This caused financial hardship. He had been a reformed vegetarian for a few years, yet still suffered repeated episodes of vitamin B12 deficiency, requiring B12 injections. He also had hay fever and seasonal asthma. Bernard's immunity had deteriorated on that diet (as did the whole family's) and he picked up every cold and flu to a severe degree. Other problems for Bernard included mental fogginess and inability to organize work activities.

My six-month-old baby Andrew seemed OK, except he hadn't put on any weight for a month and had had watery stools since birth. He had also just become himself again after his routine vaccinations at four months of age. Immediately following these he became like Harriet, overly excited and excitable, excessively loud and overactive. It was a radical personality change and I worried that he had developed ADHD.

Then two and a half years ago a friend lent me Dr Natasha's book. It was one of the most exciting reads of my life as I felt like it had been written just for us; we were such typical GAPS people. It became clear that Harriet's history of frequent ear infections as a baby (all treated with antibiotics) and full immunization status were probably connected to her ADHD and other problems. She was breastfed for 15 months, yet I had had frequent candida infections. Perhaps it was passed to her in the breast milk.

I started Harriet on the Full GAPS Diet, but fairly soon she got a gastro virus and we switched to the GAPS Introduction Diet. After a few weeks on the diet her tummy aches reduced and after a few months had disappeared completely. Her eczema cleared up in the first month. Harriet's hyperactivity had decreased dramatically by the second month on the diet, and today she is no longer hyperactive. Nor is she defiant, although that took longer to disappear. The defiance returned at times when she had been having too many sweet foods like caramelized onions, baked root vegetables, etc. When we reduced the amount of those the defiance would take a few weeks to subside, yet it always did. She rarely has a 'strep throat' now or an ear infection. She recently began to walk on her whole feet, instead of tiptoeing! This change followed the introduction of beet kvass into her diet. This introduction seemed to trigger a few weeks of severe die-off in the form of emotional 'tantrums' reminiscent of the old days. We understood that it was a detox and die-off reaction, so increased her detox baths and continued with the kvass, and after several months noticed her normal walk. We have seen the tantrums return at other times, complete with violence and screaming episodes, when we have increased probiotics, probiotic foods or when Harriet has been exposed to chemicals (such as in a renovated flat we were staying in). Detox baths and ensuring Harriet didn't get too tired seemed to help during these periods. That sort of behaviour has never been as extreme as in the pre-GAPS days though, which is a fact we have been so grateful about. The severe tantrums or emotional meltdowns decreased early on as did her unsociable, withdrawn behaviour.

Now Harriet is doing very well with her schoolwork and her ability to concentrate for long periods of time is very high. We chose to home-school Harriet for various reasons. Harriet's ability to listen has improved a lot, although that is a fairly recent development. Pre-GAPS there were no tactics that had any impact at all on Harriet's behaviour (no threat, reward or disciplinary measure). I believe she was unable to control herself, thus rendering all parental attempts to modify her behaviour completely useless. This is not the case anymore. Her behaviour can be modified. Harriet can still be impulsive at times, not looking before she leaps. There also seems to be a persistent short-term memory problem, including trouble remembering to chew her food. Harriet never used to chew her food but tried to swallow anything whole, she chews these days with a few reminders. These areas have improved a lot, yet have some way to go. I'm very grateful for this diet and the progress Harriet has made. I'm hopeful that other problem areas will continue to improve.

As for myself, I can happily report great improvements as well. I began with the SCD Introduction diet as I didn't know about GAPS Introduction Diet yet. I had severe die-off symptoms including hot flashes and such muscle fatigue that walking and talking were difficult. Unfortunately for everyone around me I was also highly irritable and short tempered. The die-off symptoms rapidly decreased after one week (although these, particularly joint and muscle pain, seemed to always be worse for me than for other people on the GAPS Diet I've spoken to).

After two months on the Full GAPS Diet I stopped losing excess hair (I had been losing my hair for six years before then!). By then my stools had become normal. My symptoms of chronic fatigue disappeared and I felt bursting with energy. I also didn't come down with a cold or flu for the last two years (I'd had very poor immunity pre-GAPS). I made a lot of mistakes on the diet that kept setting me back, so I've had to complete the Intro at stage one five times now (that has been no holiday). Some mistakes included taking *Saccharomyces Boulardii* tablets that contained lactose, and taking worming tablets that didn't contain *mebendezole* (as recommended by Dr Natasha) but *pyrantel embonate* (the active ingredient had changed since we last bought them, but we forgot to read the label). Andrew's stools were loose since the worming tablets I gave everyone. However he is currently taking bi-carb soda as recommended by Dr Natasha and his stools are becoming solid. The *saccharomyces* tablets caused my diarrhoea to return and persist for some time. The worming tablets seemed to wipe out my long-cultivated good bacteria and allowed *candida* to take over again, resulting in months of diarrhoea, extreme sleepiness and emotional overreacting. At other times my gut health seemed to regress for no apparent reason. During the times when I was free from digestive symptoms I had no asthma attacks (this has been for months at a time). As digestive symptoms have returned, so have asthma attacks in a parallel fashion. My hay fever is milder than pre-GAPS.

However, I've recently been diagnosed with the autoimmune disease Lupus. Perhaps this has been the reason behind the regressions and for my extreme die-off symptoms. Hair loss and chronic fatigue are common Lupus symptoms, yet these cleared up quickly on the GAPS diet. The word from Dr Natasha is that the GAPS Diet is the most appropriate for those with autoimmune problems, and it would appear that it is true in my case.

At present I'm not having emotional over-reactions. I feel that my reactions are normal and I can employ logical reasoning to mitigate my feelings. This is an enormous change for me and I'm overjoyed about it. Lately I've been meeting new people and haven't felt any degree of difficulty socializing (meeting new people was always painful for me as I believe I had some autistic features). My mental alertness is far greater than pre-GAPS, which I'm very happy about. One area of improvement is particularly surprising. Pre-GAPS I had made a great and persistent effort to learn to draw, but gave up after a while as I was getting nowhere and just didn't seem to be able to do it. Six months ago I picked up a pencil and started to sketch, discovering that I could suddenly do it well and it was easy! My cravings for alcohol did decrease on the diet, although very slowly, and it has only been a few months that I have been free of them.

Bernard has had no symptoms of B12 deficiency since commencing the Full GAPS Diet two and a half years ago. He has not had an asthma attack for years, despite not taking preventative medicine, whereas pre-GAPS he was quite a bad seasonal asthmatic. He suffers from hay fever to a lesser degree than pre-GAPS. His depression has never been as severe as in the pre-GAPS time, and he was able to return to full-time employment from the beginning of the diet. He hardly ever comes down with a cold or flu, and when he has, it has only been a very mild case. Bernard's depression has run a varied course in the last two and a half years, yet we've been able to track lightening or deepening of it to dietary changes, gut health and stress. At one time we ran out of Bio-Kult for one week. Big mistake! The depression deepened rapidly and didn't lessen for months. When Bernard has tried to increase his carbohydrate intake, or tried cheese and sprouted bread, or added an extra piece of fruit a day, his depression deepened. After the devastating worming tablets it deepened.

Bernard recently did the GAPS Introduction Diet for the first time, and HE HASN'T FELT DEPRESSED SINCE! He seemed to have better gut function than the rest of us, so never felt it essential to complete the Introduction Diet before.

Andrew continued to remain the same weight from five months of age. He enjoyed solids when first introduced at six months; however there was no weight gain no matter how much he ate. I increased his calorie intake and continued breastfeeding, and didn't panic as he had had a series of infections from five months onwards, and I thought that once he had sufficiently recovered from these infections he would gain weight. At seven months I panicked and made an appointment with a paediatrician. I also made a telephone consultation booking with Dr Natasha Campbell-McBride. The paediatrician's visit came around first, which was very unfortunate indeed. After talking to Dr Natasha it became clear that Andrew's failure to thrive was a GAPS condition (I wasn't really sure about the GAPS connection until then). Over the next few months I commenced Andrew on his recommended GAPS Diet and continued to see the paediatrician, at his insistence. Andrew showed some small weight gain since commencing GAPS but it wasn't enough to allay the paediatrician's fears. That Dr wanted to keep Andrew in hospital and feed him a typical diet. He went on to imply that he wasn't gaining weight because we weren't feeding him! Although many babies with failure to thrive don't like solids much, Andrew did, until about 10 months, when he went off them.

Intuitively I knew it was because his gut wasn't working properly and that when it did his appetite would return. However, until 10 months of age he ate a fair bit yet never gained weight from it. We did not consent to the Dr's treatment plan and he reported us to child welfare. He did not listen to our explanation of the diet and thumbed quickly through the GAPS book, declaring it rubbish as not many of the references came from journals he approved of. (I had been taught that the merits of any research depended on the design, method and results, not where it was published!) This battle with the Dr and the authorities and my worry over Andrew's condition were so harrowing for me that I developed heart palpitations around the clock for one week.

Fortunately Andrew began to gain weight rapidly on the GAPS Diet, and at last started having solid stools after the introduction of raw goat's milk kefir. He was 12 months old by this time. He developed a good appetite. We had delayed introducing kefir until then as he had not tolerated raw goat's milk yogurt, and we thought he had to begin with yogurt. Dr Natasha advised us, however, to try kefir even though the yogurt wasn't tolerated. He was fine with it luckily. We managed to change our paediatrician and went along to the enforced visits until Andrew was 18 months old. The new Dr was amazed at Andrew's growth rate and eventually decided that he 'should stop interfering in our lives ' (his words) as we were doing such a good job, although he didn't know how we had done it. We had not had the courage to tell him about the GAPS Diet after the trouble that disclosure caused us with the first paediatrician.

Now at the age of three Andrew is very heavy and very tall for his age, and intellectually advanced. Thankfully, the first paediatrician's predictions of a mentally retarded child, who would never reach his natural height and weight targets and may have a cardiac arrest at any time, failed to come true!

We have found the workload excessive at times on this diet (as it was on the first one we tried), feeling frequently overwhelmed by boiling pots of soup and endless dishes. A new kitchen with much more bench space helped: now I have enough room for dirty dishes and food preparation, so I can wash and cook at the same time. Harriet has recently decided that cooking is more fun than watching T.V. and so helps quite a bit! (Did my guardian angel put a spell on her?) We make this a fun time, listening to music and chatting a lot. So all in all, the workload is more manageable than it once was.

Bernard and I have discussed where we think we might be today without the GAPS Diet. We can't get away from the vision of jail for me (with my tendencies to snap and lose it) and institutional care for the rest of them! Andrew perhaps would have had part of his diseased bowel removed. When we remember where we were headed, we stop complaining and just shut up and continue cooking!

A comment from Dr Natasha

What a poignant story! This family has indeed saved itself by simply changing their diet. Our mainstream medicine is in no position to really help in any of these situations: failure to thrive, Oppositional Defiant Disorder, ADHD, autism, autoimmunity. But your own body knows how to heal itself, and all it needs is to be fed properly.

An interesting lesson from Bernard: he never had serious digestive problems, so there didn't seem to be a need for doing the GAPS Introduction diet. However, his depression disappeared completely only after he had done the Intro diet!

This family may have some way to go yet, but the largest part of their journey to full health has been accomplished. And as a result they are already a happy and successful family! Thank you, Anne!

25

Jeni

Key words: PANDAS (Paediatric Autoimmune Neuropsychiatric Disorder Associated with Streptococcal infection), PANS (Paediatric Acute-Onset Neuropsychiatric Syndrome), food allergies/intolerances, OCD (Obsessive Compulsive Disorder), anxiety, tics, allergies, urinary problems, kidney problems, overuse of antibiotics, digestive problems, reflux, eczema, reactions to vaccines, poor immunity, GERD (Gastro-oesophageal Reflux Disease), overweight

Our journey through autoimmune illnesses: PANDAS/PANS

Due to lack of awareness in both parents and doctors and for all the misdiagnosed children, I felt it was urgent to write this document and bring awareness of the autoimmune disease PANDAS / PANS. Yet another autoimmune illness striking our children! For a complete list of autoimmune-related illnesses please visit: http://www.aarda. org/research . You will be AMAZED at how many 'new' autoimmune illnesses affect our population in our current times!

Until my dietary changes, I spent my whole childhood and most of my adulthood catching every sickness under the sun. Reoccurring strep throat, bronchitis, pneumonia, colds, flu, fevers and just weird who-knows-what-bizarre illnesses!

As a baby, I had severe acid reflux and episodes of projectile vomiting. I was put on heavy duty medication that ended up being recalled! At 11 months, I came in contact with a family member who tested positive for Hepatitis B. I was given IVIG injections.

As a child, I ate SAD (Standard American Diet). My mom did cook as she knew how, using seasoning packets containing chemicals (including MSG) and meals coming from a box. I ate a ton of sweets and junk food. It was normal for me to drink Kool-Aid, Pop, and Juice, no water. I ate an abundance of fast food multiple times a week. I was on birth control pills since I was 12 due to intolerable menstrual cramps and acne.

Starting in high school I was in and out of weight watchers during my early teens and adulthood! I would have to starve myself to stay thin, never satisfied after a meal, always wanting more and struggled to fight off the horrible sugar cravings. I spent my whole life dieting and worried about every pound on the scale. It consumed me.

I suffered from stomach aches as a child. As an adult I always had Tums or Pepcid in my purse.

I had horrible allergies. The only medication that worked was Benedryl, which would leave me in a zombie state of mind throughout the day, all of spring, summer and fall.

As a child, I was diagnosed with Epstein Barr (autoimmune disorder in the herpes family), which led to a severe case of Mononucleosis in high school. I had a poorly functioning immune system and always got sick. I accepted this as a 'life sentence' and as a fact that I will always be sick.

As an adult, I lived on a low fat, high carbohydrate, high sugar diet (because that's what was contained in the fake foods I was eating). I lived on Lean Cuisines thinking I was making a healthy choice. I drank a TON of diet pop containing artificial sweetener and skim milk; again, thinking this was a healthier alternative to the regular pop and full fat milk. I was on countless antibiotics and medications to treat the various frequent illnesses I acquired. I had precancerous cells on my cervix that required a cone biopsy.

I literally 'thought' I was healthy despite being sick all the time! I thought it was just 'me' and that I had a weak immune system. I relied HEAVILY on doctors and prescription medications. Back when I worked for a company, I literally used all of my 'paid time off' for sick days, NOT vacation.

This was my 'normal' life. I didn't know better!

Fast forward to my pregnancy and the conception of Calei:

I did get pregnant easily, and now I know, given my health, that was a TRUE miracle! However, from an immune perspective, my body could not handle being pregnant and pretty much shut down. This was it; the straw that broke the camel's back sort of to speak. So many things take place in your body when you are pregnant. My weak immune system could not take the strain and biological demands of being pregnant.

First, I was miserable from the day I conceived! I remember my wonderful husband buying me a book called *Pregnancy SUCKS!* I literally had EVERY symptom in the book! The list was endless!

After conceiving, I immediately got a cold that led to bronchitis and pneumonia and lasted about eight weeks – two months!! I took Nyquil, antibiotics, cough medication with codeine, Advil, you name it, despite it not feeling right in my gut! I was told by my doctor that it was okay to take these medications while pregnant! If I only knew better!

After the sickness passed, the horrible symptoms continued. By month two I was getting unexplainable right rib and spinal pain. This led me to permanent bed rest by month three and for the remainder of my pregnancy due to excruciating pain. I could not sit or stand at ALL! I had to lie flat and rotate ice packs on my ribs and spinal area. I was given Vicodine daily for the pain and was told it was fine to take during my pregnancy. Again, if only I'd known better!

I was sent to an infectious disease doctor who ran a bunch of blood work only to find out nothing. It was probably some uncommon autoimmune/hormone issue sparked by pregnancy. My hormone levels were in the high twin range but I was only having one baby. The doctors didn't have a clue. I suffered terribly during this pregnancy!

The Birth of Calei and on...:

I went into premature labour which was stopped with more medications.

Due to my intolerable pain, Calei was born one month early via elective c-section. She weighed 6 lb 9 oz but was born with jaundice. She had issues with her liver from day one. Also, thrush (yeast overgrowth) from day one! She spent the first week in the hospital.

My bizarre, rare nerve pain DID subside after delivery! Recovering from the c-section was a breeze compared to the nerve pain! We thought the nightmare was behind us.

I began to breastfeed Calei at the hospital but due to feeding issues

I was told to supplement her with formula! Again, only if I'd known! Most formulas contain corn syrup, hydrogenated fats, and synthetic vitamins that the body cannot even use! At this point, I was still consuming a Standard American 'toxic' diet. She was diagnosed the first week of her life with GERD (Gastro-oesophageal Reflux Disease) and was put on acid reflux medication.

We took our beautiful baby home. Her feeding issues escalated to violent vomiting episodes. Not just a little spit up, I mean a TON of vomit projecting out of her little mouth! We saw a specialist and she was put on a heavier duty GERD medication (Prevacid) twice a day! We were told to have her sleep in her swing and that she would eventually 'grow out of it'. Again, if I'd only known!

At six weeks, we found her in the middle of the night soaked with puke and lifeless. The vomit was dripping from her swing. She was burning up. We immediately brought her to the ER. They ran a boat load of tests including a spinal tap and due to her age and symptoms they admitted her quickly. With lab work, the docs determined she had an unknown infection, one kidney had shut down, the other one was not functioning properly and she had a large cyst in her bladder. She had immediate surgery to drain the cyst. She was put on heavy duty medications to keep her alive. The side effects of these medications were downright scary, but had to be done. She had a 50/50 chance of living. Later we learned that she had four ureters (these are the tubes that connect your kidney to your bladder). Normally you have only two. We learned that these ureters were refluxing, meaning her urine would exit the kidney, go through one of the ureters, try to get into the cyst-crowded bladder and reflux toxic waste right back up into her kidney, hence causing kidney damage. We would learn that she would need extensive surgery around 18 months to correct the problem. Calei spent one month in the hospital, then was released, and then relapsed and spent two more weeks in the hospital. At three months we finally brought her home! Due to the above, breastfeeding stopped at six weeks and she was strictly on formula. She continued to have severe reactions to the formula. During this time we tried all sorts of formulas: cow milk, soy milk, etc... She ended up on pre-digested cow milk formula (Alementum). At the end of the day, no formula worked! Not ONCE did a doctor or nurse suggest a milk intolerance or allergy.

They sent Calei home on long-term antibiotic (Bactrum) and Prevacid twice daily. The antibiotic was to prevent infections until she was old enough to have surgery. Little did I know I was KILLING her immune system! Not to mention, her diet was fuelling the fire!

Once home, Calei continued to be a very sick baby. She caught everything! She had reoccurring ear infections, colds, coughs (including croup), you name it! Not to mention I caught everything she got! She had bad allergies and eczema. We were always at the paediatricians getting countless stronger antibiotics! I looked back at her records and she was at the paediatricians about every three weeks with some kind of illness. At one point, she had scarlet fever. Later I would connect the dots when it came to PANDAS.

I was always sceptical about vaccines, but at this time because she was SO SICK the docs convinced me that it was all the more reason to vaccinate! Again, if I'd only known! Literally one month after being released from the hospital she was vaccinated (multiple vaccines at the same time). She got these cocktails at month 4, 6, and 8 to 'catch her up'.

Calei's reactions to the shots were severe. Her paediatrician said I was overreacting. At that point I took pictures and videotaped her after receiving vaccines. She was limp, lethargic, high fever, diarrhoea, and her eyes would roll back in her head! NOT NORMAL! Yet when I showed the paediatrician the video and pictures she seemed shocked and said she never saw a reaction like that.

Calei got all her vaccines except MMR and Chicken Pox (because, due to these reactions and my prior understanding of vaccines, I began to read ALL I could and came to the conclusion I made a TERRIBLE mistake vaccinating her!) I have learned so much about vaccines since then. I would choose to NOT vaccinate, especially on a sick baby! I also look back at the health of the staff at the doctor's office. All the women were very overweight and their kids were always sick, yet they were giving me medical HEALTH advice?

Calei had surgery on her urinary system, after which she was not recovering well and was readmitted to the hospital. She had a high fever and was not clotting internally, a complication in about 1% of all patients. Another sign that her little body was not able to do what it was supposed to do, given all the trauma both in the womb and since she was born. Two blood transfusions and more medications later and we knew she'd turned the corner. From there forward, and for many many reasons, we began referring to her as the 1%.

Up to this point, for the first two years of Calei's life she had your typical American Baby diet (SAD Standard American Diet) on top of countless medications too many to list here! Rice cereal was added to her diet as an INFANT to 'help' with her reflux and to help keep the food down. Later, I learnt how much grains aggravate reflux! The only thing rice did was make her fat! She was a huge baby! Again, people thought that was 'cute'. It's NOT! She did not like baby food veggies; she just wanted baby food fruit. She was super, super picky! When eating solids she ate barely any foods! She ate: Kraft mac and cheese, McDonald's chicken nuggets (she would gag at a hamburger), McD's fries, spaghetti, and applesauce. This list is disgusting! I didn't know a limited diet is a clear sign of allergies and a very toxic system! She was always hungry too! As if she was not absorbing what she ate. I would later come to understand about malabsorption and malnourished children.

Once this was behind us and Calei was recovered fully we decided to take her to Children's Hospital to finally address her severe allergies. She was always sneezing since the time she was a baby. Everyone thought it was so cute. It's NOT. She always had this rash around her mouth and would have bouts of eczema.

I told the allergist that I had noticed when she ate a Blue Dum Dum sucker (corn syrup, food dye, sugar) she would get a rash. I was laughed at! And was told no way could that be possible! I am not kidding. Laughed at! I told them Calei was leaking urine and I think it was due to what she ate. They told me she was distracted. Calei has always been developmentally ahead of the curve, way ahead, so I knew my child and she was NOT distracted!

They did a skin scratch test and determined she had bad seasonal allergies and NO food allergies! I left there with FIVE prescriptions for my two-year-old! One to put on her skin, one to shoot up her nose, one for her ears, one for her eyes and oral Clariton. THAT WAS IT! As I left the doctor's office I threw them ALL out in the trash can at the door.

Between my pregnancy and ALL of her stuff up until this point I'd had it with Conventional Docs! I knew in my gut there MUST be another option to get us healthy. I began reading and reading and reading non-stop and reaching out to healthy people. Sad to say, I only had two healthy people in my circle of friends and the rest came from books, and online resources.

This is where I say it's a journey BIG TIME! I felt like we turned a corner and began climbing this huge mountain. I was 100% committed to the journey and determined to find answers to our health problems. But believe me, it was NOT easy. What to read? Who to believe? EVERYTHING I had been taught was being questioned! Everything I had been taught I realized was WRONG! Meanwhile, Calei and I continued to be so sick, catching everything, and dealing with our coughing, sneezing, runny nose and allergies. The clock was ticking.

A whole year went by! Yes, a WHOLE YEAR from when Calei was two to three years old, gathering information, sorting through all the information. It was very uneasy and overwhelming to take control of our health. I was so brainwashed to think DOCTORS are in control of your health! Boy was I WRONG!

Please note, there IS a time and place for doctors, especially in life or death situations. For instance, if we did not have the docs when Calei was six weeks old she would NOT be here today! BUT day to day, healing your body and knowing HOW a body works, YES, we ALL need to take control of that piece!

Gratefully, I fell into the hands of a naturopath named Barbara Griffin. Barbara sensitivity tested Calei and me and we got a clear picture of the foods we needed to avoid. Sure enough, both Calei and I tested super sensitive to corn syrup, food dye, wheat, dairy and many other specific foods. As I thought, Calei was highly sensitive to the melons that were causing her to leak urine, but fine with all other fruits. (Once we removed melons, she stopped leaking urine!) She was not distracted, as the allergist previously indicated!

We made drastic changes once we had this information. We cut out all that we were sensitive to and replaced them with gluten-free, dairy-free options. However, I call this stage of our journey the 'gluten-free dairy-free junk-food diet' high in sugar, carbs and processed grains. While we did make health gains we certainly were not eating 100% 'healthy', yet. We were still consuming an abundance of all those expensive processed gf/cf foods and lots of grains. We still ate out including fast foods but chose gf/cf options. I still consumed diet Coke and 'fake cream' in my coffee.

During Year 1, my life-long allergies were under control by taking a supplement called Quercertin. This was the first year of my life I was not drugged up on Benedryl for months! Calei's rash went away. We were not as sick as we used to be.

I began to notice that if I 'cheated' I would feel awful! By the end of this year, if I cheated, I would have violent reactions. Within four hours of consuming the food I was sensitive too, I would begin to tremor, vomit and have diarrhoea for about 12 hours. This reaction happened numerous times until I finally stopped cheating!

I have since learned that once you eliminate what you should have not been consuming and you add it back in ('cheat') before truly healing internally, your body will not tolerate it! It was clear in my case what my body would not tolerate.

The biggest improvement came in year two. We began eliminating gf/cf processed foods and moved to more of a real food diet. This process was gradual. We still ate out occasionally but we were becoming pickier where we ate. We bought organic meat and eggs from the store (but from grain-fed animals). I was trying hard to eliminate diet Coke and 'fake cream'. We still consumed sugar.

We saw more significant changes. For me, the thing I noticed the most was effortless weight loss. My allergies were gone with no supplements! This was incredible! This was the FIRST season of my life I was able to ENJOY spring, summer and fall without carrying around a box of tissues! I never had nice nails and this year they started to grow! I noticed that Calei's tastes were changing and she was trying and enjoying more food now than ever!

We also began to remove toxic chemicals in our immediate environment. I researched healthy alternatives to chemical-based soaps, cleaners, lawn care, etc...

Year 3 was even better! We eliminated corn, potato and most all grains except for an occasional slice of millet bread, and we eliminated SUGAR! Once again, for me, I effortlessly lost weight. I also noticed an abundantly sustained amount of energy. My sleep patterns changed. I never slept through the night and now I'm going to bed early and waking early.

We stopped eating out and chose to eat home-cooked meals instead. I mention eating out because along this journey I was shocked to discover that even at high end restaurants, the quality of food was awful. For example, I learned that so many places do not even carry REAL butter but some concoction of butter-like spreads. It was almost impossible to find grass-fed organic meat anywhere! We joined a local co-op and were able to get quality organic grass-fed free range meat and eggs from a local farm. I learned that if the animals were consuming corn, grain etc... that you too were consuming those if you ate the meat and eggs from them.

Calei was doing fabulously, rarely EVER sick, allergies gone, and all the other medical issues, gone! But I knew we were not out of the woods. To heal an immune system that is damaged takes years for some! That's the truth.

Calei develops PANDAS

When six years old Calei was cognitively advanced for her age, creative, and a humanitarian at heart. She was a grounded, centred child, beyond her years. Therefore, given this information, the following 'symptoms' I am about to present are totally out of character and unlike her. For instance, some children are hyper, she is not. Some children lack judgement, she excels in this skill. Some children forget what they are told (short term/long term memory), she remembers everything.

Calei got a bad cold in December 2011 that lasted a week. She also had a sore throat in January and February 2012. Nothing major, but sometime around January symptoms began to emerge. Like a slow, snowball effect, we saw a three-month decline in who she was.

In February-March Calei developed an 'open mouth' tic: she would open her mouth wide. Then she developed a 'whistling' tic: she began whistling, at first occasionally, but by February it was constant. The mouth tic also became constant. By April Calei turned into a 'picky eater' not liking the foods she LOVED just a few days ago. She developed short and long term memory loss: I caught myself repeating to her over and over to follow an instruction like washing hands. This was extremely disturbing as this skill for Calei was solid: she retained information like a genius before. Calei normally loves to read, play piano, do home school, take care of our cat, and model/act. Within the blink of an eye, she didn't want to do anything – almost a depression-like symptom. She only wanted to do gymnastics. However, I clearly saw an obsessive attribute to her gymnastics. She would do handstands and cartwheels NON-STOP. She developed more tics: slurping up her saliva and a sniffling tic. She has always bitten her nails. Now however, it was intense, almost like eating and picking her fingers to the bone, sometimes causing them to bleed! OCD-like symptoms appeared: I noticed she would flip between being SUPER messy and hoarding, to extreme cleanliness like organizing her crayons by colour. She started doing odd behaviours that even as a toddler she never did. For instance, she was colouring on furniture, she was slamming doors repetitively, she went to touch a pot of boiling water to feel the steam. I could go on and on with a list of odd behaviours. This was so out of character for Calei. Usually her judgement is that of an adult, always making good choices. She developed separation anxiety and became hyperactive. Calei is the most independent child I know; separation anxiety is foreign to us. It began at night, being afraid to fall asleep, afraid to be alone. She was over the top hyper at night, jumping on the bed, uncomfortable in her own skin. We eventually moved her mattress into our room and she slept next to us. She would say things like "I NEED you", but I was literally right there. It was as if she wanted our bodies to merge together. I noticed she was going to the bathroom more frequently. She also wet the bed (Calei was potty trained at 18 months). People who know Calei begin to notice a 'change': she had become very hyper, she could not attend, focus or stop whistling in class. She began regressing back to being a baby/toddler. She would do 'baby talk', ask me to do things like getting her dressed or brushing her teeth. She suffered severe acid reflux as a newborn and toddler. With dietary changes, this was at bay. However in the month of April, it came back.

To an outside observer, who didn't know Calei, she looked just fine. Tics, yes, but some of her tics like whistling blended in. Her hyper behaviour accepted because well, 'she is only six'. However, as her mom, who knows this child backward and forward, I knew this was not normal for Calei. I was watching her slowly deteriorate right before my eyes. I remember at some point in all this saying to my husband, 'she is beginning to look autistic!' There were subtle behaviours, little things that one can only notice from being around children with autism for 17 years like myself. Thank goodness for that experience. Therefore the pit in my stomach grew even bigger. Awful anxiety and had feeling inside. I worked with hundreds of parents of children with autism with similar stories. They would explain how their child regressed right before their eyes. They would share how their doctor would 'rationalize' the child's behaviour as 'normal', 'not to worry'. For instance, the child would be labelled as a 'late talker', 'going through a stage', etc... The fact is, the regression might look different at 18 months vs. six years, but it's the exact SAME problem!

Some trigger happened (vaccine, illness like strep, etc...), then invaders got in the gut, took over, penetrated the blood brain barrier, and attacked the brain, causing mild to severe symptoms and all in between. Due to Calei's fragile immune system and weak genes (we get sicker each generation with our current lifestyle!) she has been diagnosed with yet another autoimmune disease called PANDAS (Paediatric Autoimmune Neuropsychiatric Disorder Associated with Strep). However, the new name will be PANS (Paediatric Acute-Onset Neuropsychiatric Syndrome) as many kids are presenting with the same 'symptoms' NOT strep related, but some other 'trigger' that causes inflammation.

The treatment

Medical treatment for PANDAS is experimental. Many kids with PANDAS are misdiagnosed and put on antipsychotic drugs for TICS and OCD which do NOTHING to treat the core problem. This is an OUTDATED 'band-aid' approach. Typical PANDAS treatments are antibiotics, ibuprofen, IVIG, steroids, etc. With my daughter's damaged gut, and less-than-perfect liver, I just didn't see the above as an option! I had to find an alternative to support and boost her immune system, not wipe it out! Plus, I became part of many PANDAS support groups. I listened carefully to what was helping children 'recover' from PANDAS. Most kids saw amazing gains with the above BUT it was short term! We were looking for a long-term fix not a band-aid quick-fix approach.

Calei and I started a treatment, which I named the Calei Clark Protocol: the first army in line was our diet. We follow GAPS (Gut and Psychology Syndrome, Campbell-McBride) diet 99%. I say 99% because GAPS is very individual. This is how we got to the point of eliminating our allergies and constant sickness, among many other health benefits and being medication-free. Our diet is as clean as a whistle, nothing added to feed pathogens (sugar, carbs or grains). Lots of foods added to KILL pathogens (home-made broth). I believe over-all, that we had an advantage over beating PANDAS due to our clean diet. I cannot imagine if we were dealing with PANDAS on a Standard American Diet!

Our next army of defense would be Colloidal Silver Hydrosol, George's Aloe Vera Juice. We also took three heavy duty probiotics: Prescript Assist, Renew Life and Theralac. We also used a variety of antibacterial, antimicrobial, anti-inflammatory essential oils primarily to help reduce inflammation

We love David Wolfe! At the perfect time an email came in my inbox from him about taking control of your health using power of mind. So timely! We watched the video together and like an instant transforma-tion I saw Calei gain a confidence over PANDAS like never before! I can't emphasize ENOUGH empowering your child. When new symptoms emerged, I would say, "Calei, remember this (behaviour) is NOT you, it's the bad bugs, remember, they are NOT allowed to attack your brain, go take five minutes alone and tell them to leave!" It is also so important to help your child remain calm and comfy as best as you can during those extreme episodes of OCD/Anxiety/TICS etc... Coaching them verbally and non-verbally. For example, reminding them to simply breathe.

Connecting and Grounding with Earth: this was HUGE! I noticed an incredible decrease in behaviour when we were hiking in the woods, surrounded by nature and at times with shoes OFF! This was just as important to her as any supplement or diet! We would sit under the willow trees by our pond in our backyard and just 'be'.

And here we are now! We are still on the road to recovery to heal-ing our gut (immune system). This can take up to five years or more depending on the person. Given our history, we are pretty damaged. We are both still working on digestion and absorption. Many of my organs were severely impacted due to many years of poor lifestyle habits, all of which is passed along to Calei. Given Calei's history of the first two years of life her organs are also affected. I will know I have achieved great health when my liver begins to work properly and my acne subsides. I will know Calei is healed when her bowels are consistently healthy and, knock on wood, we don't hit any bumps in the road. This is the best year yet.

The point of my story is that if I knew back then what I know now I am 99% sure my pregnancy would have been FINE! I was too unhealthy PRE conception! Depending on how sick you are, it takes one to five years on a truly clean diet to get healthy, to clear out toxins, and build a strong immune system, strong enough to handle conception, pregnancy and post pregnancy, among many other things. It takes a TON of dedication, determination, faith and knowledge on the individual's end to venture down this path. You must have a strong desire to take control of your health and chuck most of what you have learned up to now. There have been days I have questions that go unanswered or bizarre detox-like symptoms that have no explanation. But when the time is right I am provided with answers and affirmation that I am on the right track for long-term health.

I rely so much on intuition to guide me in the health decisions I make for myself and my family versus searching outward for answers. I am grateful every day for research, the internet, my ability to learn, my support network and my faith. I will never ever stop speaking about this information I have learned. HUMAN BEINGS CANNOT LIVE ON FAKE FOOD, CHEMICALS AND BE INJECTED WITH NEUROTOXINS AT BIRTH WITHOUT PAYING THE PRICE. Period! Common Sense! It's time to go back to REAL nutrient-dense food, chemical FREE living pre-pregnancy, so that we can produce HEALTHY children!

A comment from Dr Natasha

PANDAS / PANS is a fairly new diagnosis, and indeed many doctors are not familiar with it. Typically children develop symptoms of OCD, tics, learning and behavioural problems out of the blue. Because streptococcal infection has been found in a proportion of these children, it has been initially blamed for the disorder. But the problem is deeper, Jeni is absolutely right! The problem is that the child's immune system is not functioning well, the gut flora is abnormal and the gut wall is damaged. Further research will show that not only streptococcus is implicated in PANDAS but many other pathogens, and the toxins they produce. Thank you for this poignant story, Jeni!

Jeni runs realnutritionblog.blogspot.com where she documents Calei's and her progress in the treatment.

26

J.B.

Key words: PDD-NOS (Pervasive Developmental Disorder – Not Otherwise Specified, this diagnosis is often given to non-typical autistic children), eczema

Peter was diagnosed with PDD-NOS in the fall of 2007 at three years and three months of age. We started gluten-free, casein-free diet around November 2007. We started Eva's (Peter's sister) dietary intervention around March of 2008 when she was only 11 months old, by weaning her earlier than we had planned from breast feeding and starting her on the cleaned up diet her brother was already on. We started the SCD in the summer of 2008, and then began GAPS in the fall of 2008. We saw huge improvements every step along the way as we cleaned up their diets. We were just coming to the final stages of the Intro GAPS diet in the summer of 2011. We have gone VERY SLOWLY but have found great healing. Peter has recovered and Eva will never have an ASD diagnosis, despite the fact that she exhibited many early symptoms. We've also cured her raging eczema. In addition to dietary changes we implemented very selective, super-clean (no binders, fillers, additional ingredients) DAN protocol supplementation, OT, PT and extensive ABA.

My children were very lucky to have a family that was so up to the challenge of figuring out autism recovery. I have a degree in molecular biology. My science background has allowed me to figure out some of the science required and to use the scientific method to analyse and observe the kids as we tried new therapies, diets and foods, one change at a time. My late husband James, who passed away in March of 2009, had an elementary education degree which allowed him to sound the first alarms regarding Peter's development, deal patiently with his symptoms and struggles, implement ABA at home and work with Peter through many of his challenges. My parents have been overwhelmingly supportive. As parents of five children themselves they brought a wealth of patience and parenting skills to bear. My Mom also has a parent coaching degree. My Mom's understanding of the concept of whole foods, home management skills, and cooking ability are the ONLY reason that we've been able to come so far on the GAPS Diet. The extended family has stepped up as well with support in many different ways. My children are very lucky to have them all.

I will always remember the exact date when Peter began to recover. Not because I made a note of it mentally at the time. Not because my life was or is so calm and serene that it's easy to remember minutia. But because the large wall calendar we used to scribble down family appointments at the time still hangs in my bedroom, showing the month of December 2007. There, next to doctor's appointments and bill payment deadlines, in James' handwriting are three notes about Peter's behaviour written over the course of less than a week.

Sat. Dec. 8th – Peter told/made first joke.

Dec. 11th – Peter is playing with stuffed animals. Talking to them! Having them talk to each other and to him.

Dec. 13th – Peter and James had three-sentence conversation about football in the kitchen.

No big deal. Standard behaviour for any three and a half-year-old. But new to Peter, who at the time had no original language of his own (his speech consisted entirely of scripting and echolalia), demonstrated little recognition of the nuances of social interaction and rarely used toys for anything other than stimming (self stimulatory repetitive behaviours like lining things up, or moving them past his eyes, or placing them one at a time in a box and then out of the box and then in the box again). James was the primary caregiver. A devoted dad. Tuned in to his kids. And he recognized, despite the stress and exhaustion of caring for Peter and his infant sister, that what he was seeing was a turning point. A moment significant enough to warrant stopping and noting the day. This was the awakening. The beginning of the end of the symptoms of autism that had been blocking Peter from the world around him, from us, from what he wanted and needed and desired.

The truest first sign of recovery was Peter sleeping through the night. I don't have that date written down. It was probably within the two weeks before the first note on the calendar, definitely within the month before. I remember that it was day four and five of our early stumbling efforts at dietary intervention. Our sad first attempts at gluten and casein free. But that small dietary change was enough to make a difference. We saw the improvement and knew for certain then that healing was possible for Peter and that diet would be a huge part of it.

I remember that it actually got worse in some ways as we saw larger and larger glimpses of Peter through the 'fog' of his symptoms. We would see great moments of clarity, communication and development, and then it would be back to the struggle. Knowing what he was capable of, who he truly was in there, made the set backs hard. And then the moments came when he had recovered so much that we saw his recognition of the struggle. We saw his reaction to slipping back out of control. It became emotionally more difficult when we knew for certain what he wanted to do and say. When we knew that it wasn't that he wouldn't do it, but that he couldn't do it. And saw in his eyes the recognition that something was wrong, that he had lost control. Terrifying!

I remember an incident when he came into our bedroom early in the night and wanted to get into bed with us. I wonder when this was. Six months later? Maybe only three? We talked to him. Told him that he could. But he didn't. And he didn't. He stood there and talked with us, and moved back and forth on the sides of the bed. He talked to James and then to me, asking the same questions over and over. He began to cry. We talked with him. Told him to take a deep breath, decide what he wanted to do and do it. We grew impatient. It was late, and we'd been through this before. We grew quiet and waited. It was hard. Either one of us could have gotten up and got him. He may have run away then, upset, or joined us happily in the bed. But that wasn't the point. He needed to do it himself. We all waited. He grew quiet, stopped pacing, but began to shake. We could see and feel him struggling. No doubt in anyone's mind what he wanted. Long, long moments went by. And then, finally, Peter won. Somewhere a dam broke and he ran to the bed and climbed up between us, crying hysterically, inconsolable for minutes and then happy that he was in our arms. We both cried too as we took turns congratulating him, trying to sound moderately calm and casual. "Hey you did it!" "Great job, bug." "You did what you wanted!" We had seen him fight this battle everyday over a million little things and loose. He was beginning to win. He was recovering. But the struggle was painful to watch. James and I stared at each other wide eyed as Peter drifted off to sleep between us, spent. And I remember James saying over and over, "God, that was awful!"

Those days are long behind us now. We still have grumpiness and negativity on bad days. If something with his supplements gets super messed up he can hesitate or go back and forth, just for a few seconds while making decisions. Normal indecisiveness that could be seen in anyone, especially any six-year-old. But I know what it truly is. I have seen it before. And while it's overwhelming to think that we may all struggle to keep it at bay for the rest of his life, I find strength in the fact that Peter is winning. And I am so glad that James was there to witness those early days of victory.

I hope this encourages and helps to motivate. Like I always say, while GAPS can be difficult, logistically challenging, and expensive, it is NOT MORE difficult, logistically challenging, or expensive than caring for a child and then an adult who is still suffering from the symptoms of autism. Thank you so much for your work!

Our best update right now is the glowing data we received from Peter's reevaluation by our school district. This school year, Peter attended a mainstream classroom and only received extra assistance with Speech Therapy. Academically, Peter is well advanced of what's currently required of him and he exhibits no major problem behaviors of any kind. He does still struggle with some of the finer nuances of social interaction and he shows impatience when the class is working as a group, (he prefers to hurry through an assignment in the hopes of having time to draw or read). To summarize by quoting from his IEP report, "Standardized testing and checklist results indicate no needs in regards to cognitive skills, academic skills, sensory processing, occupational therapy or social emotional functioning. Needs are still present in the area of pragmatic language and social skills." We still have areas to work on, but this report shows SO MUCH success and victory for Peter, his teachers, his ABA tutors, his speech therapists and his family! This report indicates what we already knew, that in four and a half years *Peter has almost completely recovered from all his autism symptoms!* An AMAZING feet, accomplished despite the death of his father.

Now, in the summer of 2012, we are still taking the last steps in the final stage of the GAPS Intro Diet. We have successfully introduced almond flour and we are looking forward to the upcoming baked goods. Our next major step will be fermented grains. We have not moved through the diet and onward in two years as we may have once hoped. But the children still seem to be quite sensitive, and we are greatly motivated to keep them functioning at their very best every day. We have never hit a complete road block and we will continue pushing forward no matter how small the steps need to be.

The children are enjoying their summer vacation. Their swimming is just taking off and Peter is biking, training wheel-free. We are exceptionally busy, but I still strive to get information to families who don't yet know that recovery is possible, as well as those who don't know where to begin. I started a facebook page called *Off The Spectrum*, were I post the links that have been the most helpful for us (GAPS diet, ABA, etc.), so other families can then scroll through at their convenience.

I am grateful and beyond optimistic for these happy, healed, capable, caring, calm, loving, bright and brilliant children who are interested in everything and everyone around them, who sleep through the night, and who roll with the many changes in our goofy life. Their smiles are the best part. These children smile all day now. Not just when you tickle them or when they're watching a funny movie, but all day long as they move through their lives. A hard fought victory! And worth all the effort!

A comment from Dr Natasha

Thank you very much for your story, J.B.! It is difficult for people, not familiar with autism, to understand what it is like to hear your child speak correctly, make decisions or do anything else 'normal'. And it does take the whole family effort to heal a child from autism. Thanks to that Peter is doing well. As the family got on track with healing Peter, they managed to save his baby sister from the same fate. I am sure that both the children will remember their dad as a person who helped them to have normal and healthy lives.

ADULTS

1

A.

Key words: vegan / vegetarian, irritable bowel syndrome, endometriosis, PMS, infertility, anxiety, extreme reactivity to stress, insomnia, heart palpitations, iron-deficiency anaemia, underweight, postnatal depression, miscarriage, inflammatory arthritis, vaginal thrush

Dear Dr Campbell-McBride,

I want to give you my heartfelt thanks for having restored my health with your GAPS Programme!

I'm a naturopath in Australia.

I'm now 37 years old and for the last 10 years my health has steadily deteriorated, despite my best adherence to widespread naturopathic regimes (generally high fibre, low saturated fat, high in whole grains and protein, fresh fruit and vegetables).

In my 20s I embraced vegetarianism for health and, particularly, the well-known acid-alkaline diet. At first I felt great but this only lasted a couple of months, followed by the onset of SEVERE IBS (Irritable Bowel Syndrome) and worsening of menstrual symptoms. My cholesterol level plummeted to 1.5 and I was told that this was very healthy and obviously a reflection of the pure diet I was on. Meanwhile, our efforts to conceive were not successful and I was diagnosed with endometriosis.

Severe digestive trouble plagued me daily, and I experienced agonizing bowel pain and increased urgency nightly. This was followed by the onset of free-floating anxiety, extreme reactivity to stress, insomnia and palpitations as well as unresponsive iron-deficiency.

It was not a pretty picture. My health improved somewhat once I reintroduced animal produce (lean protein at the time), some probiotics and demulcent fibre. However, my nervous system was shot and for years I relied on naturopathic herbs and supplements to keep me going. Any amount of stress would make me feel extremely anxious and teary and this was obviously exacerbated in the last days of luteal phase.

After having my daughter I became very depleted and lost a lot of weight. No matter how much I ate, I couldn't keep the weight on. I became severely exhausted and eight months after the birth succumbed to postnatal depression. In the meantime, vaginal thrush became a regular occurrence and I was advised by my then naturopath to increase fish and soy and avoid all meat as I was oestrogen-dominant.

So I started eating fish and soy daily – often I would eat a whole packet of tofu in one sitting as I felt hungry all the time. My naturopath enthused about how healthy my diet was, with incredibly high amounts of vegetables, beans, whole grains, berries and phytoestrogens (!).

Through herbs and rest I overcame the depression, however my digestive system was seriously compromised despite taking daily high-strength probiotics.

So you can imagine my surprise when, a year later, I was rushed to hospital with emergency appendicitis. I felt I'd been deceived! I couldn't understand how my colon could be in such bad shape when I had the 'best' diet of anyone I knew.

Then I started researching and started speaking to an amazing naturopath, Angela Hywood, who exposed me to Weston A. Price precepts. Boy! What a learning curve that was. Everything I'd learned in naturopathic college, professional courses and personal indoctrination went out the window! However, my digestion was too far gone to transition straight to WAPF. I experienced a miscarriage and that was my turning point for leaving all nutritional DOGMA behind!

After my miscarriage, I developed severe ongoing bilateral joint pain. Various investigations left doctors puzzled as I didn't show any arthritis markers but there was obviously a lot of pain and inflammation. I developed a bony spur in my left, fifth metatarsal-phalangeal joint which was perfectly palpable and swelling in both hands.

I started searching WAPF more in depth and, finally, while looking for a recipe for sauerkraut that didn't include whey (I'd become dairy

intolerant) I came across *GAPS Australia*. That was it! As soon as I
started reading about GAPS, I had a Eureka-moment. I was very familiar with your descriptions of digestive physiology and bacterial flora
but your treatment of leaky gut and healing of the villi and their
involvement in disaccharide digestion just blew me away!

I set out to follow the programme religiously. The first two weeks on
the Intro were hell. Linda Paterson at GAPS Australia warned me that
I might experience die-off symptoms, but in my blinkered view I
couldn't quite admit to myself the extent of my dysbiosis – heck! I'd
spent a small fortune on practitioner-only, high strength probiotics for
years!

Well, let me tell you... .Even with doing baby steps in the
programme, I experienced such exhaustion and flu-like symptoms that
it really brought home the message: I was on a fast route to major
intestinal issues unless I sorted this out!

Regular colonics helped a lot and bit by bit my energy came back.

To cut a long story short – I'm now a different person! My husband,
sceptical at first, doesn't recognize his wife anymore and so he's started
the GAPS programme too. That's another story but to make it short –
his insomnia is cured; he no longer carries excess weight round his
middle and has bags of energy despite a very stressful job.

These are the benefits I'm now experiencing:

- best digestion I've had in 10 years;
- no more pain – ever;
- zero PMS;
- no more pelvic congestion in the week before the period;
- high resistance to stress – even under great pressure;
- great sleep;
- steady energy throughout the day;
- I can't remember the last time I felt anxiety or palpitations;
- no more thrush;
- after an initial period of losing weight on GAPS I'm now back at a
  healthy weight and not super-skinny anymore;
- the bony spur I developed a year ago is almost all gone – making
  me understand how impactful a treatment this is for anyone with
  inflammatory arthritis.

I know that my health troubles were small compared to the many families with children on the spectrum the GAPS Programme has helped, but I wanted you to know that I'm so grateful to you! I believe you've given me (and my family) a second lease of life! I'm so in awe of this Programme that I'm going to do the training to become a GAPS Practitioner next month. I see many mothers and fathers-to-be who would benefit greatly from following GAPS.

A comment from Dr Natasha

Thank you for your letter! It demonstrates how pervasive nutritional misinformation is in our modern world! Plant-based, low-fat, high-fibre and vegetarian diets have been touted as healthy by mainstream for years. So many well-educated and intelligent people fall prey to this propaganda, with dire consequences to their health. It is a typical pattern to feel well on these diets for the first one to two months, because they allow the body to cleanse. Of course, a cleaner body feels better than a body full of toxins. However, plant-based diets do not feed the body to any extent, they only cleanse. So, once the body has finished cleansing it becomes hungry, very hungry. This is the point when you need to start feeding your body with animal-based foods, because these are the 'feeding', building foods, which provide the body with 'bricks and mortar' to build itself from. If the person continues with a plant-based diet beyond that point, the body enters a stage of true starvation and becomes ill. Please read more on this subject in 'Feeding versus cleansing' on my blog: Doctor-Natasha.com.

2

Tara

Key words: Crohn's disease/Ulcerative colitis, anaemia, diarrhoea

The GAPS Diet ended a six-year nightmare for me and gave me my life back!

In the fall of 2009 I was desperate for a miracle. I had been living with severe Crohn's disease/Ulcerative colitis for five years and, at 30 years old, I found myself wasting away with the disease, living from one hospitalization to the next. I couldn't eat ANYTHING without immediately getting sick. I was a prisoner in my home, unable to leave for fear of not being near a bathroom. I was in daily excruciating pain and having bloody diarrhoea, sometimes up to 18–20 times a day. The constant bleeding was so bad, I became severely anaemic and nearly lost my life on a couple of occasions due to shock from blood loss; my haemoglobin had dropped so low.

I had been on every medication available to me: Asacol, Budesinide, Flagyl, Prednisone, and 6–MP. I even spent six weeks on TPN (Total Parentheral Nutrition). I was hospitalized and fed through an IV only (intravenously). The hopes were that the bowel rest would trigger some remission. But as soon as I began eating again, my gut would cramp painfully and relentlessly and I'd be running for the bathroom. Finally, it was suggested that it was time to try Remicade, 'the miracle drug.' I had been putting it off, as I knew the severe and very scary possible side effects. With no other options, I relented and underwent a full round of Remicade in August of 2009... The miracle drug did NOTH-ING. It didn't even stop the bleeding. I cried as my gastroenterologist told me that she was sorry but there was nothing else she could offer me except surgery. I felt so beside myself, I thought that it might be time to face the music – to accept the fact that I would remain in this

161

living hell for the rest of my life, unable to date, get married, have children or a career – things I acutely longed for.

During this whole nightmare, I had tried several alternative therapies. Having a natural interest in health and nutrition prior to my diagnosis, I was becoming an 'unofficial expert' in the field. I was always researching and looking everywhere I could for answers beyond medication, as I knew this wasn't the answer to truly heal my disease. I tried several months of acupuncture, chiropractic, NAET therapy, herbs, different diets, fasts, etc. The therapies would sort-of keep me afloat, but the right treatment, the 'silver bullet', eluded me.

Through a series of events that I have no other explanation for, except Divine intervention, I was led to a gal who worked for Dr Thomas Cowan in San Francisco. She told me that Dr Cowan had had success with treating Crohn's with the use of Low Dose Naltrexone (LDN) and a special diet. I was sceptical, I had tried so many alternative therapies; and at this point I was living back at home with my parents and was flat broke. But I recognized that I was out of options. Why not get one last opinion? The alternative would be going under the knife – something I was adamantly opposed to.

Two weeks before Christmas 2009, my mother and I went to my appointment at Dr Cowan's office. He listened to me for 45 minutes; he wanted to know my whole health history. In all of the years that I had Crohn's/ulcerative colitis, he was the first person to be able to tell me what was going on in my body, how it got that way, and what I needed to do to reverse it. He prescribed the GAPS Diet, which I had never even heard of. But when he explained how it worked, it made so much sense! It was like the sky had opened up. I remember walking out of the office into the daylight; my mom and I looked at each other almost in disbelief. This new concept, this diet, seemed to hold so much promise. But we had been through so much; there was still scepticism in the back of our minds. We recognized it would be a huge commitment, and at the end of the day we wondered, *"Could the GAPS Diet really be the answer we've been waiting so long for?"*

I went home and read the book, and while it was absolutely enlightening and fascinating, it was overwhelming! It took me two months to research and practise and learn about the diet online, there were so few resources at the time. I finally felt ready to give it the old college try, and on 15 February 2010 I began the GAPS Intro.

I went extremely slowly, probably too slowly through the stages. I was so very ill I was afraid of doing too much too soon. The first week I felt great. I had good energy, did journaling, and worked through my fears of not having grains. The second week, however, 'die-off' began to hit, and it hit hard. I came down with the flu: sore throat, fever, cold, cough and, to my terror, bloody diarrhoea. I was crushed! I thought it was a sign that the diet wasn't working and that it had been too good to be true. I immediately got on the GAPS online forum and got encouragement and help. I practically lived on that forum for the first several months! It took about three full weeks to get through this massive sickness, but after which, I noticed, the bloody diarrhoea disappeared and my tummy was becoming calmer and calmer.

At about a month and a half, I had the hunch that this diet might really be working. I was not worse for wear, and I did really feel nourished, had more energy, and my daily pain was gone. There was a period at around two months where my bowel movements sort-of went through this 'adjustment stage.' I began to experience some constipation for the first time, but used the protocols, the enemas and worked through them. After a while of this, my bowel movements became more and more consistent, solid, formed. Pain and bleeding were a thing of the past. At about three months in, I would turn to my mom and say, almost afraid to jinx it, "Mom, I think I'm getting better". And she would reply, "I think you are too!" We were almost afraid to even say it. We were in disbelief that this could be working after years of such torment. People began to make comments about me having a 'glow'– even people who didn't know about my illness.

About five months in I was ready for home-made kefir. I had gone through the six-week elimination of dairy and slowly reintroduced it. Anxious to try this highly lauded food, I received some kefir grains from a dear friend, dropped them in beautiful raw organic milk and gave it a go. I quickly fell *in love* with it! It was like my body just craved the stuff and I couldn't get enough. I drank several glasses a day, plain or in smoothies and all of a sudden, I didn't have to wonder if I was getting better – I KNEW!

In September of 2010, it had been seven months since beginning the GAPS Diet and I was absolutely floored to find myself completely free of any Crohn's or UC (ulcerative colitis) symptoms! I realized that just a year prior, I was facing the Remicade infusions and now here I was, experiencing a bona fide miracle that wasn't tied to any drug. I was overwhelmed with joy and relief!

Two months later, I took my last weaned dose of the Crohn's drug (6–MP) without even a bump in the road; my body had become so sturdy and strong. That was in November of 2010. I have been completely drug-free and symptom-free from Crohn's ever since...

I remained on the GAPS Diet 100% and completely strict for exactly one year total. After that, I became more lax, began to experiment with incorporating grains once again. To my delight, I found that I handled them just fine and could even eat 'forbidden foods' on occasion, like pizza or ice cream, without a problem. These days, I eat a variety of whole foods, grains in moderation (many of them properly soaked and prepared, but not always). I still like to eat fermented foods, home-made kefir, bone broth, sauerkraut, etc. when I can. I will always keep these amazing foods in my diet. I still do the protocols on occasion, like detox baths and juicing. But now I can enjoy a meal out, or eat at a social gathering and not have to stress out. I consider GAPS as my baseline – it's a foundation I use to keep my body in balance and to promote health. Overall, I would say that my diet is very much based on the Weston A. Price principles and is always changing, based on my intuition, my current needs, the season, and so forth. At the end of the day, no matter what my diet, I no longer battle Crohn's. It's just gone!

I can't tell you the gratitude I experience on a daily basis. This diet absolutely saved me and enabled me to live my life again. In the fall of 2011 I made the decision to return to school for holistic nutrition. Living through what I did, I knew that I had to share my experience and do my best to spare others the suffering that I once had. I am now certified as a Holistic Health Counsellor and have the opportunity to 'pay it forward,' share my experience, educate, and let people know that true healing is possible. It's astounding to me how things have come full circle. My desire is that my story will act as a beacon of hope and light to those still battling in the trenches of pain.

I want to stress that I'm not 'lucky', or 'special'. My story is not a fluke. The truth of the matter is that the GAPS Diet was exactly what my body needed to heal. I can't possibly know what your body needs to heal, but if you feel that the GAPS Diet resonates with you, I highly encourage you to give it an honest try. The path to healing may not always be identical but we must hold on to the truth: that there are answers and solutions for the modern epidemics that we face. If we all work together to seek these answers and solutions, we can reverse the tide of health crisis and create a world where we eradicate disease. I challenge you to take a leap of faith and join in!

A comment from Dr Natasha

Thank you, Tara, for this wonderful story! I am sure that it will help many others to recover from Crohn's disease and ulcerative colitis. I strongly believe that there are no hopeless situations, and that there is nobody out there beyond help! And you have confirmed this belief once again. Thank you for that!

Tara runs a website www.metamorphosisnutrition.com where you can learn more and get in touch with her.

3

Ashley R. Hathaway

Certified Nutritional Therapist, Certified GAPS Practitioner

Key words: digestive problems, food poisoning

Over the last few years, I have heard my fair share of GAPS stories, so I know mine is really not extraordinary. However doing the GAPS Diet was one of the more profound experiences of my life, and that is why I want to share it.

In late 2009 I had a rather acute gastro-intestinal illness that I thought would simply need to 'run its course'. In the couple of years prior, I had several bouts of what I thought was food poisoning – and looking back, I think this may have been part of the breakdown of my gut health overall. After several weeks of unbearable acute symptoms, I found myself with my first opportunity to seek help from Dr Thomas Cowan.

When Dr Cowan first moved his practice to my neighbourhood (Glen Park in San Francisco), I wrote a story about him for the *Glen Park News*. During my interview with him, he gave me a copy of his book and this sparked my interest about the way he practices medicine and the *Fourfold Path to Healing*. I then found myself looking into the Weston A. Price Foundation and Sally Fallon.

Not wanting to see my primary care doctor at UCSF for the conventional medicine route to figure out what was going on in my gut, I called for an appointment with Dr Cowan and he was able to see me that week. He examined me, asked a series of questions, and along with ordering a faecal test to rule out the possibility of a nasty invasion of *salmonella, shigella*, etc. he explained and prescribed the GAPS Diet. Walking out of that appointment totally overwhelmed and curious, I began a full-fledged research mission to figure out what the heck this GAPS Diet was about and what the difference between a disaccharide and a polysaccharide was!

I began the GAPS Introduction Diet the very next day and followed it to the letter (no pun here!) for the next four months. Eight days into the diet I began to feel relief from my horrible symptoms. After about 40 days, I was feeling 100% better, although not all of my symptoms were gone.

I have to say, the GAPS Diet was one of the hardest things I have had to do in a long time. And to make it even more difficult, my first 30 days on it just happened to fall over the Thanksgiving holiday and I was doing the Full GAPS through Christmas and New Year! Not fun.

After four months, I began incorporating some dairy and soaked grains into my diet and after eight months, I was 100% symptom-free and eating a Nourishing Traditions diet. I also joined the WAP Foundation and found myself telling my story over and over to all sorts of people with surprising results.

To date my symptoms have never returned... and not a single bout of 'food poisoning' or GI upset!

After this experience, having already had a fair amount of knowledge about healthy foods and diet, I realized that I had learned much more than I ever would have imagined about the digestive system, and using food to heal the body. This experience was so profound for me that I decided to quit my freelance career of 20 years as a video producer to pursue a certification as a Nutritional Therapy Practitioner. I received my NTP certification in June 2011 and in addition, received a GAPS Practitioner Certification in September 2011. I now have my own practice called *San Francisco Nutritional Therapy* and a website www.sfnutritonaltherapy.com Through my practice I find great satisfaction in helping others achieve wellness using whole foods, natural supplements and, when necessary, the GAPS Diet.

A comment from Dr Natasha

Thank you for your story, Ashley!

GAPS Introduction Diet is the best way to deal with any food poisoning or any other gastro-intestinal infection, acute or chronic.

This diet will sooth and heal the gut lining quite quickly and permanently. Depending on how long the problem has existed, it may take from a few days to a few months to heal. For example a child who picked up a 'tummy bug' at school can recover in only a few days, while a person with Ashley's situation will need several months.

Ashley indeed has qualified as a Certified GAPS Practitioner in autumn 2011 and is running the San Francisco Nutritional Therapy centre. You will find her contact details on the Find GAPS Practitioner page on www.gaps.me.

4

Shann Jones

Shann Jones is a farmer. She supplies wonderful organic raw
goat's milk and kefir from her farm in Wales, UK,
www.thechucklinggoat. co.uk

Key words: ulcerative colitis, goat's kefir and raw milk

When I first met my husband – a vigorous, hard-working, outdoor-
loving farmer – he had severe, steroid-resistant ulcerative colitis. The
colitis was under control at the time with the help of infliximab, a
powerful drug for which he reported to the hospital every eight weeks,
and received intravenously over a four-hour period.

But over time, the infliximab gradually ceased working, and the
colitis returned. I watched with dread as he came home each day
increasingly grey and exhausted with pain. The nausea, cramping
and blood loss were unrelenting. The accompanying rheumatoid
arthritis in his joints became more and more painful, and he shuf-
fled across the yard like an old man, although he was only 47.
Caring for the dairy goats and sheep on our farm became a frightening struggle.

Determined to find a solution, I began to research. Working
together with the hospital, we went through every solution that
modern medicine could offer. One of the drugs we tried was so strong
and so expensive that it had its own funding string from the government, and was delivered to the house in a special van every two weeks,
with its own injection system.

But nothing worked.

Finally, we organized a referral to a world-renowned colitis specialist in London, who was doing some innovative work in the field. We
went to see him full of hope. He told us, very gently, that we had

exhausted all the possibilities, and that the next stop was a colostomy. We went home devastated.

And then the very next day, just as we were about to make the appointment for his surgery, *my husband went into remission.* All his symptoms just disappeared. It was like a miracle!

What had caused it? We had no idea, but we were so grateful for the miracle that we didn't question it too much.

Then we heard Dr Natasha Campbell-McBride being interviewed on the *Food Programme* on Radio Four, speaking about raw milk. It was the clearest scientific explanation I had ever heard. We listened with fascination, because for the last two years we had been producing and drinking raw milk from our own little herd of dairy goats.

Because we had so much surplus milk, I had also been making home-made kefir, which my husband had been drinking. And because we butcher our own lambs on the farm and freeze them, I make a lot of meat stock and soups, because simmering the big lumps of meat (with the bone in) in water, is the best way to cook them.

In other words, I had been feeding my husband the GAPS Diet increasingly for two years, without even knowing it!

I ordered the GAPS book straight away, and read it cover to cover. Finally, everything made sense. Rich's miraculous remission from ulcerative was no miracle, and no coincidence – it was a direct result of the fact that he had been eating the GAPS Diet!

During that time, my five-year old son had also been completely cured of asthma, eczema and troubling bronchial infections. In fact, my entire family had gotten incredibly healthy!

My husband has been in full remission for a year now. And my eyes fill with tears of joy whenever I watch him working around the farm, full of radiant health, slinging heavy hay bales, pounding in fence posts and wrestling with the sheep!

Inspired by our very own personal miracle, I slogged through all the horrendous red tape required to become registered and licensed to sell our own raw goat's milk, in its active form. I succeeded – and we are now legal to sell raw goat's milk. It was the toughest thing I've ever done – those government people sure didn't want us to do it! But it is legal in England because they have failed to ban it (as they did in Scotland). We plan next to get approval so that we can ship and sell the frozen raw goat's milk online. And we're also going to be producing fruit smoothies made with raw goat's kefir – which is surprisingly unknown and hard to get hold of in this country, and which seems so much more powerful than yogurt! We hope to make these products available online to other people who are struggling as we did, to make it easier for them to achieve their own miracles!

Thank you for your work, Dr Natasha! It is really, truly, deeply life-saving!

A comment from Dr Natasha

Thank you, Shann for this lovely story! It just shows that good health can be created on a natural mixed farm simply by following your instincts and rationality.

Milk of any animal (including humans) is the female's white blood (with red blood cells removed); IT IS ALIVE! It is made from alive and active immune cells, antibodies, probiotic bacteria, active enzymes and hormones. It is full of nourishing substances in their natural active form: proteins, fats, carbohydrates, minerals and vitamins. When we pasteurize milk we kill it. We destroy the immune cells, the antibodies, active enzymes and probiotic bacteria; we change the chemical structure of proteins, carbohydrates, fats, minerals and vitamins, making them difficult to digest and be of any use for our bodies. Drinking pasteurized milk loads your body with dead polluting substances, which your body has to work hard to dispose of. That is why pasteurized milk is the number one cause of allergies, digestive disorders and autoimmune disease. There are hundreds of scientific studies showing that pasteurized milk products may cause cancer, heart disease, diabetes and every other common malady in our modern world. None of that applies to the raw milk, straight from the animal. On the contrary raw milk is known to help in curing allergies, digestive disorders, autoimmunity and many other health problems. Shann is supplying raw goat's milk and kefir from her organic farm in Wales, which can be ordered on her website www.chucklinggoat.co.uk

Thank you, Shann, for this service to humanity!

5

A.S.

Key words: digestive disorder, malnourishment, low body weight, anxiety, insomnia, antibiotics

I've been on a long journey ever since I was needlessly prescribed two rounds of antibiotics (one of which was broad-spectrum), when I was misdiagnosed with a bacterial sinus infection (discharge was clear, so not bacterial). That left me with a constant burning in my chest, and I was severely underweight and unable to put on the pounds no matter how well I ate. My GP was no help as he prescribed two different PPIs (proton pump inhibitors – drugs to reduce stomach acid), each giving a worse allergic reaction. I then followed treatment options from a Naturopath, and a couple of holistic MDs. I've had great success with them.

However, I noticed most treatments avoid some foods that may aggravate a compromised digestive tract, and provide supplementation. What really excited me about GAPS is the complete elimination of all such substances, and the emphasis on foods proven to heal the digestive tract and rebalance gut flora. It truly is the most comprehensive protocol I have encountered (and researching this stuff has become a BIG part of my life, ever since I got sick).

So, it was with much enthusiasm that I started the GAPS Diet, underweight and stuck at 145 lb (up from a low of 137 lb), but in high spirits from previous progress attained through natural medicine. I was truly amazed that within two days I had gained 4 lb, and within five days I had put on 6! It seems all of a sudden my body started properly absorbing nutrients and that quickly accelerated my path to recovery. I've continued on the diet – it's been about three weeks now – and I feel better than ever. I haven't weighed myself in a few days, but I believe I continue to gain!

I'm 6ft 2 and my weight before getting sick was about 152 lb. I was probably chronically underweight most of my life (typically close to 145 lb as an adult). I got pneumonia in grade 4 and was hospitalized. Ever since then I can recall being a very picky eater, as you describe in your book. I basically only ate refined carbs, cheese, lunch meats, sweets, and would not touch vegetables! I've always been very skinny. However, I've always excelled academically, although I can often remember feeling as if I had 'brain fog'. I had some aggression issues and got into some fights as a kid.

So, it's possible I've been suffering from dysbiosis for most of my life, but didn't have serious digestive issues until this latest round of antibiotics. Preceding this incident I had severe anxiety for years, mostly social. I also had insomnia for years. My only digestive symptoms were heart burn, especially after eating curry or drinking red wine. However, a few months before the antibiotics I tried the candida diet for a month. When I went off the diet I had a sudden change in the shape, consistency and smell of my stool. It's at that point that I saw a gastroenterologist, who scheduled me for a colonoscopy. After I got sick from the antibiotics, we added an endoscopy and did both... while I was in the midst of my most severe dysbiosis. All tests came back negative. The one test that I believe did show something was the organic acids test that I ordered from Great Plains Lab.

I'm continuing on the diet and my only symptoms are constipation. I have two or more eliminations per day, but usually at least one is hard and requires straining to accomplish. I eat meat broth with soft boiled eggs at almost every meal, along with sauerkraut 10 minutes before. I'm also using organic yogurt and kefir. I buy the yogurt, kefir, and sauerkraut from health food stores. I know you recommend doing it home-made, but it's difficult for me to find the time. I'm buying what I believe to be very high quality, organic products. I haven't been able to follow the Intro Diet, as I'm very busy with work. I would like to follow it over the holidays. I'm wondering if it's necessary, considering my symptoms are not severe.

Otherwise, I just wanted to thank you for the amazing work you're doing! There's a dire need to balance digestive flora in this generation, otherwise it seems like the health of our children will become progressively worse.

A comment from Dr Natasha

Thank you for your story, A.S.! You are absolutely right: there is a dire need for making people aware of gut flora and what it can do to the body, when it is damaged. And as the parents pass their gut flora to their children, the situation gets worse from generation to generation. The testimony to that is growing epidemics of learning disabilities and physical illness in our children.

Many people with abnormal gut flora are unable to digest and absorb food, so they are underweight and malnourished. I am delighted that GAPS allowed you to start healing your digestive system. As a result you started digesting and absorbing food properly, so now you are gaining weight and building a strong healthy body!

6

Aaron Falbel

Key words: digestive disorder, chronic cystitis, chronic sinusitis, malabsorption and low body weight, hypothyroidism, anaemia, elevated homocysteine, elevated lipids and cholesterol

I was born in 1961, six weeks prematurely. My birth weight was 3.3 lb/1500g and I lost some weight after that, going down to 1390g. In those days, the doctors gave me a 50-50 chance of survival. I made it. I was placed in an incubator for about six weeks. Consequently, I was not breastfed and was raised on some sort of formula (probably Enfamil).

Both my mother and my grandfather (her father) have had digestive problems for as long as I can remember. Especially in times of stress, my mom would get diarrhoea and have to take a pill (Lomotil, I believe) to relieve it. My grandfather's digestive problems were worse, but I don't really know the details. Late in his life, at the age of 86, he developed the autoimmune neuromuscular disease known as myasthenia gravis. For the last seven years of his life, he had to take prednisone, which, miraculously, he could tolerate. He died suddenly at the age of 93 of a heart attack. My grandfather always had something of a sweet tooth (he grew up in Vienna, after all) and my grandmother was a phenomenal baker. Enough said!

I was always a skinny child. I was underweight from the very beginning! I could not seem to gain weight no matter how much I ate. Yet I otherwise seemed healthy, so my paediatrician told my mother not to worry about it. Perhaps I had a super-efficient metabolism, he suggested.

Around 2003, when I was 41 years old, I started to notice certain digestive abnormalities. I would have to urinate quite often and with urgency. This would come and go. I'd had a prostate exam and urine analysis, which were normal, so I knew it wasn't that. I suspected it was food related, as the symptoms were worse at certain times. I suspected dairy products (milk and yogurt), tomatoes, or oatmeal as possible problem foods.

Things got steadily worse. I would frequently have loose stools or diarrhoea, gassiness, and urinary frequency/urgency. Sometimes I would have to get up five times or more during the night to urinate.

I always thought my diet was a healthy one. I ate lots of organic vegetables, whole grains, and occasionally fish or chicken. I did not eat red meat. For a while during the 1990s, I ate tofu fairly regularly. I stopped eating it entirely in 2002 when I read material from the Weston A. Price Foundation of the possible harmful effects of unfermented soy products. I never ate many sweets, and rarely had dessert, except on special occasions. I did make my own whole wheat sourdough bread on a regular basis. I studied briefly with renowned baker Richard Bourdon, and my bread got to be almost as good as his (by his own attestation). I probably ate too much of it.

I more or less lived with these symptoms, since they were not always present, but they did worry me. In 2007, I stopped eating oatmeal for breakfast, and that helped somewhat. My doctor ran some blood tests in 2008 and this revealed borderline hypothyroidism (TSH = 4), mild macrocytic anaemia (enlarged red blood cells), elevated homocysteine, and elevated lipids/cholesterol. (The HDL level was high as well, so he said he wasn't concerned about the lipids.) Having read the work of Dr Kilmer McCully, I was concerned about the homocysteine. My doctor prescribed synthetic levothyroxine (T4) for the thyroid and megadoses of B vitamins for the anaemia and high homocysteine. Neither of these medications had any effect on my major symptoms. I was losing weight, which was not good. I convinced my doctor to discontinue the thyroid medication because it didn't make me feel any better, and I didn't really have any of the 20 or so symptoms typical of hypothyroidism. I kept taking the B vitamins.

Meanwhile, my own research revealed a possible link between *candida albicans* overgrowth and hypothyroidism. The more I read about candida, the more I became convinced that this was my underlying problem. It explained all my symptoms and the results of the blood tests. In late 2009, I adopted the anti-candida diet promoted my Dr William Crook in *The Yeast Connection*. This diet allows certain grains (quinoa, buckwheat, amaranth, and millet). I did not see much improvement. In February of 2010, I obtained a copy of Dr Campbell-McBride's book, *Gut And Psychology Syndrome*, and I learned that candida rarely acts alone, and that, very likely, other opportunistic pathogenic flora had taken up residence in my gut. So I adopted the GAPS Diet and protocol, starting with the Introductory Diet described by Baden Lashkov in her *GAPS Guide*.

I had a somewhat bumpy start. A rash of some sort broke out on my face, which I presumed was a die-off reaction. I was hungry all the time and was losing weight. I am 180cm tall and my 'normal' weight was 138 lb/62.6 kg. My weight went down to 125 lb/56.7 kg and I could feel myself growing weaker. It took me a few months to fine-tune the diet and turn this around. I reasoned that when you take away all those carbohydrates in the form of grains, potatoes, beans, etc., you have to replace them with something. Neither vegetables nor protein would make up for all those missing calories. The obvious solution was to increase my consumption of fats. I never subscribed to the low-fat diet craze, and I thought I was already eating a decent amount of fat. But without those carbohydrates, it wasn't enough. *Our culture is so fat phobic that we really don't understand what ENOUGH FAT means. IT'S MUCH MORE THAN I EVER THOUGHT!* I started eating a lot more cheese (8 oz/225 g or more per day) and used a lot more butter. I also started eating red meat again, which I had not done since I was a teenager. As a result I started gaining weight and energy, and I wasn't chronically hungry anymore. Now, in January 2011, I weigh 147 lb/66.7 kg, which is more than I can ever remember weighing. I hope I will gain more weight still.

Aside note: in recent months, in *Wise Traditions*, there have been letters from people saying, like me, that they were growing weaker on the GAPS diet. I wonder if they were really eating enough fats. Dr Tom Cowan recommended adding some starches back into one's diet. I'm inclined to disagree with him. I don't think that would have worked for me.

I am not out of the woods yet. I am still sensitive to sweet vegetables such as carrots, beets, butternut squash, or tomatoes. And I can't tolerate fruits either, raw or cooked. Even though I haven't had diarrhoea for months, when I eat these foods, my sinuses let me know that there is still a problem. If I eat, say, carrots or squash for dinner, my sinuses become irritated and my nose starts running exactly one hour before sunrise – it happens like clockwork, every time! I don't know whether this is just a coincidence of elapsed time or whether it has something to do with a change in air pressure or moisture. Evidently, something is still living up there in the mucous membranes of my sinuses, and it responds to these vegetables/fruits.

I still cannot tolerate yogurt well, even the 24–hour kind, but hard cheeses, as I mentioned above, are fine. A few months ago, I started making my own kefir, and that REALLY helped. It has a much broader probiotic spectrum than yogurt, and it's much easier to make. (To reap the full benefits, you have to make it the traditional way, using kefir 'grains' and not with powdered cultures.) I drink a cup or so of kefir first thing in the morning with my probiotic capsules, and then another cup an hour or so before dinner. When I first started drinking kefir, I developed a mild, slightly itchy rash on my abdomen. More die-off reactions? The rash has since subsided.

All in all, my major symptoms have vanished, and I can't thank you enough for that, Dr Natasha. I still have to be careful about certain vegetables, even though they are permissible according to your list of acceptable foods. If and when I am totally symptom-free, I will be very curious to take another blood test to see whether the TSH, anaemia, homocysteine, and lipid levels have normalized (though I think much of cholesterol theory is hogwash and based on bad science). Now THAT would be something!

I find myself wondering why I suddenly developed gut dysbiosis in 2003 at the age of 41. Lack of breastfeeding as a baby? Cumulative effect of a high-carb diet? Heredity? All of the above? I'm inclined to think that stress pushed me over the edge. My job is physically stressful (I work on an organic farm). I don't own a car and travel almost exclusively by bicycle. There are other emotional and psychological stresses in my life, which in many ways are even harder to address than the physical ones. Perhaps I won't get fully well until I deal with those.

Update, August 2012: I have settled into a version of the GAPS diet that is high in fat, very low in carbohydrate, and moderate in protein, also known as a ketogenic diet. It seems to work best for me. My LDL cholesterol is still very high. Whether this is of any consequence, I am not sure. Roughly ten percent of people on very low carb diets develop *very* high LDL cholesterol, and I seem to be one of them. The cause is unclear. It may be connected with my (still subclinical) hypothyroidism, specifically the underconversion of T_4 to T_3. Or, my high-fat diet may be down-regulating my LDL receptors, resulting in a failure to clear excess or unused LDL from circulation. I hope to investigate this further. The anaemia problem has resolved itself. As long as I stick to this diet, I feel fine. If I inadvertently eat something I shouldn't have eaten, my sinuses, like the proverbial canary in the coal mine, let me know about it!

I believe my initial problem with the GAPS diet was not eating enough fat, as mentioned above, but I also had a problem with electrolyte balance. A low-carb diet causes the kidneys to flush sodium and potassium out of the body (along with water weight loss). When I replenished these electrolytes, I felt much better and this change helped to optomize my keto-adaptation — that is, my metabolism's transition to a ketogenic diet. I highly recommend the book by Drs Stephen Phinney and Jeff Volek called *The Art and Science of Low Carbohydrate Living*, which goes into these matters in detail.

A comment from Dr Natasha

Thank you for your story, Aaron! You are right: stress and emotional upheaval can and does bring physical problems. But your health history from birth is one of a GAPS person. That is why you were always underweight and found it difficult to gain weight; your digestion and absorption of nutrients was not optimal. Toxicity, generated in your gut was eliminated from your body in urine, causing chronic cystitis on the way. All your other symptoms stem from the unhealthy gut as well.

Aaron's story is very typical and quite common in our modern world. I am sure many people will recognize themselves in this story.

Aaron made a very valuable point: fearing fats has become second nature to people in the Western world, people instinctively limit their fat intake. Almost 50% of your body (dry weight) is made out of fats, and the best fats for your body come from animal foods. So eating the right amounts of animal fats is not optional for any human being, and it is absolutely essential for a GAPS person to recover. Your daily needs for nutrients are very individual, so it is vital to trust your body to get the right intake of fat. For people who are recovering from illness and who are underweight it may be quite a lot of fat: 150–200g of butter or a large piece of pork/beef/lamb fat with every meal. Only your body knows how much, so trust your senses of taste, smell, desire for food and satisfaction from food. Your body speaks to you through those senses, so listen to them. You can learn more on this subject on Doctor-Natasha.com in an article 'Feeding Versus Cleansing'.

7

Janice

Key words: lymphocytic colitis, arthritis, long-term use of anti-inflammatory drugs

I am 48 years old and work as a teacher. In early November of 2011 I developed abdominal pain and chronic diarrhoea, having to go to the toilet around nine times a day (two to three times during the night). Biopsies taken at a sigmoidoscopy revealed thickening of the bowel wall and some fibrosis, and the pathologist thought I may have lymphocytic colitis. I have arthritis in my knees, as well as a prolapsed disc in my back. So I have been taking anti-inflammatories intermittently for around nine years, and increasingly from September 2011 following further damage to my knee. I feel that taking these drugs may have caused the problem, though it's possible that I also had a food poisoning around that time.

I was offered steroids to help with the inflammation in the bowel, which I declined. Meanwhile I researched my condition extensively on the Internet and came across the GAPS Diet. I bought the book and began the GAPS Introductory Diet at the beginning of January 2012. The diarrhoea reduced immediately on the Introduction Diet. The best thing of all was that the abdominal pains ceased very quickly, as did the gurgling in my tummy. This gave me hope, so, although it was very hard work (especially holding down a full-time job and feeling very weak and anxious); I had the motivation to keep going.

Now I am pleased to say that my symptoms have completely disappeared! I can now tolerate fruit and salad and am enjoying them very much. Just in time for the summer! I am now on the Full GAPS Diet with virtually no problems. I don't miss anything from my old diet, except rice and potatoes, but I am hopeful that I will be able to eat them again in about a year.

I am so pleased that, as a result of the advice given in your book, I have been able to solve the problem without resorting to steroids! Needless to say, I have thrown away the anti-inflammatories and use regular ice for my back and physiotherapy for my knees.

I think as many people as possible should know about the GAPS Programme. It's amazing, when you get a problem such as mine and tell others about it, how many other people are suffering in a similar way. I have been spreading the word in my own small way amongst my circle! Thank you for all the wonderful insights that you have shared in your book *Gut And Psychology Syndrome*!

A comment from Dr Natasha

Thank you, Janice, for your story! Long-term use of anti-inflammatory drugs is a major cause of digestive problems such as various forms of colitis. There are many people in the world who suffer this way. Arthritis is often caused by abnormal gut flora as well. By healing your gut you can address both problems at the same time.

8

Hella D.

Key words: sensitivity to moulds, chemicals and EMF (electro-magnetic fields), anxiety, panic attacks, migraine, cyclical vomiting syndrome, digestive problems, allergies, asthma, hay fever, chronic fatigue, yeast infection

Prior to all of these health problems I had the best health of anyone I have ever known. In fact I thought I was invincible. Which is one of the reasons I have been so determined to regain that health.

In 2005 my partner and I moved into an apartment in Wellington, New Zealand. The apartment smelled like cat urine, but it had a big sunny window and was all we could afford at the time. So we moved in. We started experiencing a variety of health problems. My partner's asthma, which he had as a kid, returned in full force. I started menstruating every two weeks. I was very tired all the time and at work (I am a chef). I started experiencing disturbing images whenever I saw something that could be hazardous. If I saw a knife I would imagine it cutting me or stabbing into my eye. If I saw a wet spot on the floor I would see myself slipping in it and smashing my brains out on the floor. If I was working on the grill I would see myself suddenly tripping and landing face first on it. If I was working with an industrial mixing bowl I would see my arm slipping into it and shattering in all directions. I remember telling my friend that this was really strange for me, as usually I am quite happy at work. I figured it was from all of the florescent lights I was working under at the time, and financial stress.

Finally, after I was sick for three days – delirious, throwing up, with violent headaches – I got up and for some reason was looking at the floor near the window. I noticed a strange thing growing out of the carpet. At first I didn't recognize what it was as I couldn't believe it. But as I kept looking I finally figured out it was a couple of slimy-looking mushrooms (we have a photo). I called my partner over and he looked at it too, but also didn't see what it was at first (interesting how our brain filters information!). When he realized what it was, we knew we had to get out of the apartment ASAP. We were in a lease and our slum-lord refused to accept that the apartment was so mouldy it was making us sick. We had no legal recourse, so we broke our lease and moved out.

Before moving into our next apartment we took all of our clothes and blankets to the Laundromat and washed them with bleach. In the new apartment we were much better, but my partner started to experience night sweats which were so profuse they would wake us up at around 3 a.m. every morning with our bed and blankets completely drenched. We were sleeping on an air-mattress so we could dry it out every day, and would have to get up to sleep on the couch. Also, I was having diarrhoea permanently (I did so for about three months).

Finally my partner's NZ visa was up and we had to leave the country to be able to stay together. I got a job in Myanmar (Burma) as a chef, and my partner joined me there after visiting his parents in Holland where he came down with what seemed to be flu. When he arrived in Myanmar his flu had become pneumonia and he had to take a course of strong antibiotics. I had previously read the book *The Yeast Connection* and so we went on a strict no-carb diet. I also started taking a low dose of Nystatin and was eating lots of yogurt. My diarrhoea cleared up and we started doing better.

Towards the end of the time we were there I foolishly ate a melted popsicle in a very poor area of Yangon (Rangoon) while visiting a pagoda. Not surprisingly, two weeks later, I discovered I had typhoid and was immediately given very powerful antibiotics. Shortly after this we moved back to the United States. Recovery from typhoid takes a while in general, so I was not surprised to be so bone tired I could barely walk up stairs for months. We were staying in the Catskills of NY with my partner's folks as we recovered.

I have considered Sally Fallon Morell's book *Nourishing Traditions* to be my bible for quite some time, so we found a place to get raw goat's milk, but we were very poor so we ate a lot of beans and bone broths. I was getting migraines that would devolve into cyclical vomiting syndrome every couple of weeks, but I slowly started feeling a little bit better. After living there about a year we decided to move to Vancouver, BC. It was a very stressful couple of years where I had to shuttle between Vancouver and Seattle while waiting for my residency to come through. We were also very broke as usual, so we were eating lots of beans, as well as bone broths. I began getting the cyclical vomiting syndrome more and more frequently. I also was very sensitive to chemicals and EMFs and I think living in a city aggravated those conditions on top of all the stress we were under.

Finally, I got my residency and was able to settle down in one place. But when autumn arrived it was very wet and rained steadily for a month solid. I got incredibly sick shortly thereafter and was unable to leave my bed for about a month. I had severe haemorrhoids, by this time I was getting cyclical vomiting syndrome about every 10 days. I discovered that bentonite clay helped the condition as well as baths, and I got a hair analysis done. I had previously had hepatitis A as a child and my liver was weak and unable to handle detoxifying my body very well. I finally started getting some acupuncture and realized the room we were in had mould. My partner also experienced a worsening of his asthma at this time and would go into panic attacks as well, which was very scary. I am a trained cranial-sacral therapist so I could help him to relax and get out of his panic mode, but it was terrifying for both of us. During this whole time I didn't have health insurance, which I actually feel was a blessing as going to a doctor for my conditions would have probably resulted in many inconclusive tests and medications that would have just exacerbated my condition.

At this time my sister told me of her friend who was on the GAPS Diet and, after hearing her experiences with the diet, I decided we had better get on the diet pronto. I first spent time learning how to cook grain-free and then in February of 2010 we finally went onto the GAPS Introduction Diet. The first two weeks we ate pretty much only carrot soup made with rich bone broth and slowly added in eggs and avocados. The first month of the diet was terrible. My partner would wake up every morning with his nose just streaming and with severe allergic symptoms for about an hour. He kept saying it was just hay fever, but it was clear it was a result of the diet. We were incredibly irritable and grumpy with each other for no real reason, and my partner started to get fungus rashes on his belly and other areas, which he treated with anti-fungal ointments (we eventually found using kefir on the rashes is much more successful!). We started taking a bentonite and Epsom salt bath every night and that really helped to aid our detoxification and lessen our irritability.

We also were able to join a local cow-share group and access raw milk and make our own kefir. As a result we were able to add dairy back into our diet much sooner than we could have when using pasteurized dairy. At one point the authorities here shut down our dairy and we used organic pasteurized milk for about a week. Immediately we started to experience more symptoms, which cleared up as soon as we got back on the raw dairy.

We have now completed a year on the GAPS Diet. I stopped getting the cyclical vomiting syndrome right away, except if I got really stressed out and didn't sleep enough. I haven't had it now since last December (that was because we helped my uncle move to Oregon which took three days; we barely slept and didn't have access to our proper diet). My partner no longer has asthma or allergies at all! We have really come a long way but we know we still have some healing to do. I have a zillion times more energy than I used to, but I still get exhausted easily after stressful times, if I don't get enough sleep or if I eat something not on the diet.

Prior to going on the GAPS Diet I was getting soooo frustrated as we were eating a *Nourishing Traditions* diet (mostly) and I couldn't understand why our health kept getting worse. I really feel like I owe so much to GAPS for the healing we have experienced. Thank you Dr Campbell-McBride so much for all the work, effort and determination you have put into researching and promoting this programme. The Bio-Kult has also helped us immensely. I cannot say thank you enough times and will be forever indebted to you!

During these last few years when I have been sick and unable to hold down a regular job I created the website www.helladelicious.com which is all about food, health and traditional cultures, and I talk a lot about our experiences on the GAP Syndrome Diet.

I have recently realised that we have been living in an area very high in electro-smog (since moving to Vancouver). We are surrounded by cell towers and antenna on most sides. These low frequency EMFs amplify the effects of mould symptoms. The remarkable thing is how we have healed with use of the GAPS diet under these conditions! In the first month of being on the diet, both my partner and I had moles turn black and drastically change colour, my partner's moles started bleeding on two occasions. We even went to a doctor to have them checked. After a month on the diet we no longer had this happen, our moles went back to normal.

We had been on the GAPS diet for 2 years and in January we had stopped taking Bio-Kult, because we figured we had plenty of probiotics in our diet already. Immediately we both worsened, my partner started getting asthma again and got a cold he couldn't shake for more than a month. We immediately got back on the Bio-Kult which helped immensely.

I started researching electromagnetic fields. I grew up in Papua New Guinea; we didn't have electricity in the village I lived in until I was 13 years old. I am now 37 years old and am highly sensitive to electromagnetic fields. I finally discovered some devices created by a family of dowsers that converts the toxic frequencies into the Schumann resonance, and after a week or so of detox symptoms we are suddenly healthier than ever. We are still on the diet (the last stages of it – adding in potatoes and fermented grains – finally!) But, from the readings that I get of the EMFs in our building, I am sure that our healing process with the GAPS diet would have gone much faster if we had known about this detrimental effect of EMFs on us sooner. I am very relieved to have been on the GAPS diet; without it, I am sure, we would both have cancer by now.

I am a biodynamic craniosacral therapist and was having trouble when working in areas with lots of wireless (getting exhausted and taking on client's symptoms). I have also found that I am extremely allergic to fluorescent lights. I just want to let people know about our experiences with EMFs (electro-magnetic fields), as I think this is a very important added dimension to healing in our modern world.

Thank you again from the bottom of my heart!

A comment from Dr Natasha

Mouldy environment can cause very serious disease, particularly in a person with abnormal gut flora and yeast overgrowth. Moulds release their spores and toxic chemicals into the air, and the only way to deal with this situation is to move away from the mouldy environment. However, if the person has GAPS just moving away will not get rid of their health problems; damp cold weather, stress and typical Western foods will continue making them sick. Only by healing their gut, changing their gut flora and, as a result, rebalancing their immune system can these people regain their health.

An interesting point about raw dairy: when it was not available for a few days and this couple had to use organic pasteurized milk instead, they got ill again. But as soon as they returned to raw milk, they started recovering.

EMFs (electro-magnetic fields) are a growing problem in our modern world; we are increasingly living in an electronic 'soup', which we cannot see or hear, but it affects our health. GAPS people can be particularly sensitive, and for many it is essential to deal with this sensitivity to heal fully.

Thank you very much for your story, Hella D.! We can all learn a lot from it.

9

Gerald

Key words: celiac disease, recovery from drug and alcohol abuse, chronic depression, constipation

I had been free from drugs and alcohol for 15 years when I removed the GAPS 'illegal' foods from my diet in March 2009. Thirty-six hours later, I realised that these starchy and sugary foods had been the cause of the depression that had haunted me since early childhood, and which had continued to linger in the background during my time in sobriety. I have not spent one moment depressed in the past 33 months! It's like I can't become depressed even if I tried!

I found GAPS by the same kind of circuitous route that leads so many of us – finally – to an answer that works. *First*, using internet resources, I diagnosed myself as celiac in 2008, and my diagnosis was confirmed by a family doctor. *Second*, I got very lucky: my GI doctor told me not to follow the standard medical advice for celiac disease, which is the gluten-free (GF) diet! In his opinion, the GF diet offers only a temporary reprieve from celiac disease. He told me he sees his celiac patients return to his office after several years on the GF diet, dying all over again from the very same symptoms that had been killing them years prior.

I believed the GI doctor because that is exactly what I saw happen to my mother, diagnosed celiac in 1992 at the age 41, deceased in 2006 at the age 55 after 14 years on the GF diet. The GI doctor had the courage to disagree with the medical establishment, and he also had the humility to admit that he was not sure what the cure for celiac is, only that he was certain that the GF diet is not the cure. The GI doctor recommended that I follow a Hypo-Allergenic Rotation Diet (HARD). He said I would have to figure out for myself what truly ails me.

I followed the HARD diet for seven months, which of course was also GF, working closely with the GI doctor's nutritionist. It was a very hard diet to follow: the same four meals every four days for seven months; I can still taste some of them. After keeping a daily food diary for seven months, I concluded that it must be grains in general that are making me ill, because I was ill every day and I was eating grains every day. I would understand much more later, when I was on GAPS.

Third, I got very lucky again: a friend of my wife's introduced me to Elaine Gottschall's Specific Carbohydrate Diet (SCD). I had a hard time wrapping my head around the idea that carbohydrates could be difficult to digest. After all, table sugar dissolves readily in water whereas, some 'health experts' have told us, red meat remains in our bowels for up to 10 years ... What a lot of 'un-learning' we GAPS patients have had to do!

I accepted the SCD challenge to 'fanatically adhere to the diet' for 30 days, before making up my mind whether it was working for me or not.

Thirty-six hours later, euphoria! I could hear angels singing! The world was the same, yet everything was different. The spectre of depression that had haunted me since my pre-school days vanished without a trace! The Committee of voices stopped chattering – you know, those negative and self-critical voices that remind us of every mistake we've ever made and also constantly worry about anything that might possibly go wrong in the future. I haven't heard a peep out of the Committee in 33 months!

Instantly, I felt 'returned to myself', like I was brought back to a fork in the road at age four, where all my life since I had travelled down the road dominated and disturbed by the effects of the starchy and sugary 'Illegals'. And now I had an opportunity to travel down the other road, the road that Nature had intended me to follow!

An intuitive thought came to me: all alcoholics have GAPS too! Then another: and the drug addicts, the sex addicts, and the gambling addicts have GAPS! I didn't know how that could be possible, yet the intuitive thoughts kept coming: and the food addicts, the bulimics, even the anorexics – fat people and skinny people alike. They all have GAPS! THIS IS WHAT WE HAVE! THIS IS IT!

Anxiety evaporated. Lust was slowly extinguished over the weeks to follow. Anger cooled to the point that it could be laughed away.

At times, I wondered if I was crazy. Several times a day I would come into and out of my new mental state. I wouldn't realize that I 'had left,' but when I 'returned,' I would realize that I 'had been gone.' It was like waking up from a hallucinogenic drug. This happened several times a day in the beginning and didn't stop happening for about six weeks, yet during all this time I continued to go to work and lead a normal family life with my wife and child. I didn't tell anyone what was happening to my mental state, but I felt joyous. My wife observed changes in me. I was healing physically as well of many gut, skin, energy, and cognitive problems, too numerous to list here.

I learned about Yahoo SCD forums online and I joined one. I wanted to know that I wasn't the only person having this experience. It seemed like the forum members were largely parents of autistic children. Autism? How's that related to depression and substance abuse? I described my experience, but nobody wrote back ... or perhaps I just didn't understand how to use a Yahoo forum. But I concluded all the same that, yes, they think I'm crazy. I'm not going to tell anybody about this experience I've just had – and I didn't tell anyone for 18 months.

Fourth, I got really lucky again: a hydrotherapist introduced me to GAPS. Somehow, I had got it in my head that a professional colonic would benefit me. At around that same time I had been learning about candida on the SCD website. I had or had had a majority of the physical and mental symptoms. My SCD recovery had plateaued after seven months or so, and I remained constipated. I was looking for more answers. I decided to try colonics and try an anti-candida version of SCD.

On the hydrotherapist's bench, in the most compromising position I had ever been in my life, I told my SCD story to the hydrotherapist. She, too, was on the SCD. She seemed to know what I was talking about, and at my second visit she offered to sell me the GAPS text at cost. After the high cost of a professional colonic, I was reluctant to purchase a book I had never heard of, but there it was on the cover: P for psychology, and one of the road signs read 'Depression.' Yes! Yes! Yes! Someone out there understands! I bought the book and learned about home enemas, and for all her help and understanding, she lost a paying customer.

It never would have occurred to me that I could perform enemas at home, but the enema kit has become a fixture in our bathroom these past 18 months, and the daily enema has been instrumental in my GAPS recovery!

The three significant improvements for me in the GAPS protocol over the SCD diet are: 1) daily enemas, two) a diet high in fat, and three) fermented foods, especially milk kefir. Milk kefir had the wonderful ability to clear up residual mental confusion and anger that remained for the first few months after switching over from what was, in retrospect, a very high-sweets SCD to an anti-candida Full GAPS.

In the interim though, between the visits to the hydrotherapist and the time I began implementing GAPS protocols, I went anti-candida, and some dramatic changes took place. I experienced three rounds of voluminous diarrhoea, I who was the chronically constipated type and had rarely had a loose stool in all my life! This voluminous diarrhoea was of a peculiar consistency and had an unnatural odour, neither of which I recognized. And it was extremely painful. I was doubled over, pounding my fist against the tile floor, moaning in agony I experienced all too often since early childhood. But, after each round of this extraordinary diarrhoea, relief! And after the third round, I rapidly experienced more healing: just when I thought things couldn't get any better, they did. I had even more peace and physical healing!

I wish to reach out to my fellow alcoholics, particularly those who have shared the similar experience as recovered alcoholics who have continued to struggle with depression or other mental disturbances despite their many other successes in sobriety. I will gladly welcome correspondence from other addicts of all stripes who can relate to my experiences, and especially those who have found a solution in GAPS.

I never would have believed any of this, but I experienced it first hand. Seeing is believing! I think back to a discussion early in my sobriety, where the topic was 'alcoholism caused by nutritional deficiencies'. We all laughed at the notion. Old-timers and newcomers alike dismissed the idea out of hand; we had contempt for the notion without ever investigating it.

How things would have been different if I had heard the story of a GAPS recovery from chronic depression early in my sobriety! But better late than never, and I am truly grateful for that. After cleaning up my past and making amends for the harm I had done others, after paying back my financial debts and debts to society, after having adopted a more mature and moral attitude than I ever would have believed possible - after all was said and done, it turns out that the biggest problems in my life before sobriety had not been of my own making. Rather, they were the direct result of my inability to digest the basic staples of age-old agrarian diets: grains, beans, potatoes, and sugars, including milk sugar, all the GAPS illegals.

Like most medical doctors still today, I never recognized the now obvious symptoms of malnutrition and gut disease that I had presented all of my life, nor their relationship to the mental burdens I carried with me from my pre-school days. At my first reunion with recovered alcoholic friends after removing the GAPS illegals from my diet, however, I had to sit on my hands and bite my tongue. My gut was screaming at me. On every face and in every story, I saw the effects of this common malnutrition we share, whether we be alcoholic, autistic, schizophrenic, simply depressive, bi-polar, etc. The faces of the hundreds of recovered alcoholics I have met over the years, plus the thousands of alcoholics who weren't able to achieve sobriety, flashed before my eyes.

Erstwhile unexplained phenomena of non-alcoholic family troubles were suddenly explained: depression, obesity and other eating disorders, severe mental illness like schizophrenia! Only a minority of our family members become 'real' alcoholics, but so much of the rest of our extended family is shot through with the devastating effects of 'carbohydrate maldigestion.' This was 'it'! This is the common thread that weaves its way through the generations. This is why the '-ism' runs through our families even when relatively few of us succumb to alcohol-ism. The religious explanations failed to satisfy. Likewise, the child abuse and the 'genetic' explanations failed to satisfy. But the hypothesis of carbohydrate maldigestion is a complete answer. This is 'it'!

I came to believe that it is no simple coincidence that there is a high degree of overlap between two groups of people: 1) people who don't handle alcohol very well and 2) people who don't handle grains, beans, potatoes, and sugars very well. These foods were not consumed by pre-agrarian hunter-gatherers. We are not well adapted to them. A look at just the recent historical record, even at present day living, recent descendants of Old and New World non-farming aboriginals, shows us how both alcohol and starchy and sugary foods can devastate the physical and mental health of people not long accustomed to consuming such foods.

My own North European forebears have had a bit more acquaintance with alcohol and the GAPS illegals than have the Inuit, just to take one example. But in the larger scheme, it has not been all that long that my own ancestors have been farming and drinking alcohol. I believe that recovered alcoholics who continue to struggle with depression, for example, should give GAPS a try. I was not myself any kind of food addict, bulimic, anorexic, etc.; it never would have occurred to me that food had anything to do with my mental state. Yet my experience first on the SCD and then GAPS has demonstrated that I am one of the many human beings, who would do much better without ever consuming either one of these groups of agrarian foods.

Thank you, SCD, and especially thank you, GAPS, which I still practise today! Before GAPS, I was resigned to trudging the road of unhappy destiny for the rest of my life. Nowadays, I am completely unburdened! My new mental state has been a free gift. I did not work for it other than removing the GAPS illegals from my diet and incorporating the other portions of the GAPS protocol.

P.S. July 2012: 39 months and not a moment depressed. Still free of anxiety, lust, anger. Off anti-candida and enjoying GAPS legal carby foods with success. Have benefitted from 'extremely high' animal fats, at times as much as 25 – 30 added tablespoons of fat to my daily fare. Began Hulda Clark liver flushes and coffee enemas as per GAPS protocol in December 2011. Recently tried the GAPS iodine painting protocol to address hypothyroid symptoms and I saw results. Have since joined Yahoo iodine group and have implemented their protocol, ***WOW***, this could be another GAPS 'cherry on the top' for me. Just when I think it can't get any better, it does! I feel a strength and confidence I have never known. I feel great!

A comment from Dr Natasha

What a great story! And told with such humility and sense of humour! I absolutely agree with you, Gerald: starches, sugars and all other processed carbohydrates are the hidden cause of most chronic maladies and miseries of our modern society. And yes, when you suggest it to any uninformed person they do not take you seriously. But please, don't sit on your hands and bite your tongue anymore, talk to your friends and colleagues! Talk about your experience and your discoveries, talk without any fear! Some of them may ridicule you and not listen, but there will be others who will take it on board, and you will save their lives!

For those who would like to learn more Gerald has kindly provided a link to a radio interview: http://www.blogtalkradio.com/gapsjourney/two011/0five/twoeight/gerald—healing-digestive-disorders-on-gaps-diet

10

John

Key words: mental illness, chronic fatigue, epileptic seizures in the past, manic depression

First of all I would like to thank Peter Campbell-McBride for his time and the conscientious way he dealt with my telephone enquiry. But now I would like to give the biggest thank you I have ever given to anyone in my life to Dr Natasha Campbell-McBride! It has been barely a month since I digested your wonderful book and less than three weeks since I put your diet into practice. It has transformed my life!

After the detox period I now feel properly well for the first time in living memory. I have had a digestive disorder since early childhood, glandular fever, about six incidents of grand-mal epilepsy over six years (at the age of 18–24), hepatitis B (with no explanation of how I contracted the illness – I never took drugs or practised any unsafe sex... in fact at that time I still had not had any sexual partner), then a history of manic depression stretching over 10 years with two psychotic episodes. During this period, and especially after I had moved on from the manic mood swings (as well as phasing out the lithium medication with psychiatric cooperation), I was still disabled by chronic fatigue and mild but persistent unipolar depression.

Less than three weeks ago I started the GAPS Diet and immediately felt better. I then went through detox and felt bloody awful. But I am through that now and I feel like ill-health is just dropping off me like a reptile shedding an old skin. I am experiencing feeling well for the first time.

My ill-health has been especially difficult to bear during the last eight years since I have two children, four and seven, and I could not be the positive, energetic parent I wanted to be. Now, with my health hopefully being restored, I can enjoy parenthood and all family life to the full. You have given me this chance.

I worked for a brief period for a charity called the Family Trust based in York which gave grants to families in need with children with health problems and disabilities. It was clear that ADHD, autism, ADD, etc. were increasing at a phenomenal rate. They represented a large percentage of all the applications for grants from desperate families with heart-rending stories of what they had to cope with. Why is it taking so long for the mainstream NHS to accept the importance of diet and the science / medical research which underpin your work?

All GPs I have dealt with have been at best friendly but useless, at worst patronizing, prejudiced (against mental health) and resistant to pursuing any worthwhile investigation into my condition. I have tried exclusion diets before, but they all start with brown rice and were merely based on food intolerance... none worked because what I needed was the GAPS Programme.

You really have given me back my life... My working life has been very fragmented and my career (despite managing to graduate from Kings College London) blighted by my illness. Now I feel I am stepping out onto the stage again. I am so optimistic, quite excited, elated but with my feet firmly on the ground.

So inspired am I by your work and what you have done for me that I am considering, at the age of 45, retraining as a nutritionist. I feel you have the key to so much ill-health in modern Western society. Mental health professionals must listen - surely this could be a health revolution! But I suspect rather a lot of psychiatrists would be out of a job if your approach became mainstream. And the food industry would hate it of course...

Thank you again!

A comment from Dr Natasha

Thank you for your letter, John! What a wonderful story! It just shows that there is no medical condition or diagnosis that the human body cannot heal. As long as you give your body the right nutrition and remove toxins, it can heal anything and at any age! Somebody clever once mentioned that there are no rewards or punishments in Nature, only consequences. The epidemics of learning disabilities, physical and mental illness in our children and adults are consequences of what we, humans, are doing to our planet, our food supply, our bodies and the environment we live in. You are right: the change will not come from the authorities. But I think humanity is starting to learn the lesson, one person at a time!

11

Lydia Rose

Key words: sugar addiction / cravings, OCD, eating disorder, obesity, drug and alcohol abuse, suicidal depression, anxiety, asthma, allergies, vegetarian / vegan, migraines, amenorrhoea, PCOS (polycystic ovaries syndrome), celiac disease, hypoglycaemia, joint pain

My name is Lydia Rose, so named because of the severe rosy rash I had on my face when I was born. My background and history are completely GAPS-y. I am a GAPS adult and was a GAPS child. A friend who is in my WAPF chapter said to me, "you are the walking picture of GAPS!" I had to laugh, because it is true. Reading the book was like unlocking a key to my life. It has been life-changing just to have the information, not to mention all the changes that have come from implementing the diet.

As a child I had ear infections, yeast infections, and the aforementioned rash. I had keratosis pilaris on my arms, legs, and face and dry, cracked feet. I was also very anxious and OCD, writing and reading obsessively by age three. I always had food issues – I would get 'food poisoning' at least 10 times a year and threw up quite a bit. At age five I started having uncontrollable sugar cravings and would awaken in the middle of the night to find myself eating frosting off a cake or handfuls of brown sugar. I could eat bowls and bowls of pasta and could then throw it up just by thinking of it; my stomach became so full and distended. I started wetting the bed and woke up with debilitating leg cramps. I became severely overweight almost overnight at age five, and my food cravings continued to plague me. Noodles and cookies and cereal I could eat and eat and eat. I was always hungry but never full.

I was clumsy and when I broke bones they didn't heal, creating large cysts around them instead. We had skim milk, which made me gag, and I developed severe tree nut allergies at age six. My stomach always hurt and after meals I would have to lie down and push up hard in-between the bottom of my ribs in order to even breathe. I decided to become a vegetarian at age 12, because I couldn't digest meat. I stayed a vegetarian until I was 28.

By the time I was in junior high I weighed over 200 lb. I wrote obses-sively and became an insomniac. I started craving cigarettes even though I had never smoked, and started doing drugs. I also craved marijuana and started smoking it all the time.

I developed bulimia. In high school I fluctuated between anorexia and bulimia. I became compulsive about languages and art, often stay-ing up for days learning extra languages and finishing art projects. I was extremely compulsive and started stealing things even though I didn't need to.

I became a vegan because just being a vegetarian wasn't helping my stomach, and because I wanted to lose more weight. I lost about 100 lb and then crashed. I wasn't able to walk or even concentrate in school and became suicidal. My periods stopped. The doctors put me on a heavy dose of Paxil and Trazodone, which made me fuzzy. I took a year off from school and my weight started to climb up even with the severe restricting and exercising. One thing I always felt was that my body did whatever it wanted with regards to weight and I couldn't stop it. I felt like I was swinging from one end to the other, no matter what I ate or did. My stomach would puff out and my head would become noisy. My sugar cravings became worse as my medicine was increased. I woke up eating jars of jam or bowls of cake batter at 3 a.m. in the middle of a sleep-eating episode. I weighed 100 lb at age 18, and 235 lb at age 19. I had migraines on a weekly basis that sent me to bed – these migraines continued until GAPS.

I started doing more and more drugs, and especially drinking. I was a blackout drunk almost overnight. I went to college and got straight A's, but my world was splitting apart. I lost another 75 lb and started having concussions because I could get drunk on so little alcohol. I started cutting myself. I had been slapping myself and pinching myself for as long as I could remember, but now I felt compelled to cut my skin. I started having seizures. I was splitting apart. I took myself off all my anxiety and ADD drugs and antidepressants and had a suicide attempt. I was in the hospital for three weeks and then went to the psychiatric ward. I weighed 90 lb and refused food.

After my suicide attempt my drinking went downhill. My college kicked me out for my suicide attempt. I continued my drinking for a few years, along with bulimia, gaining and losing 60 lb, and then got kicked out of two more schools. I had intense food cravings and stole food and alcohol compulsively. Finally, I woke up in an alley one day and decided I needed treatment. I went to treatment and almost got kicked out for drinking gallons of juice that was meant for the whole group and snorting sugar. Yes, you heard right. I needed sugar so badly I snorted it! Eating handfuls of it did not seem to be enough! I became addicted to diet Coke and would drink 24 in a day. I lost weight again so I was around 100 lb. My bulimia raged on, but I stopped drinking and remain sober to this day.

After being sober for around a year I started to gain weight almost overnight. In a month I gained 40 lb. In six months I weighed 200 lb. I started to grow a little beard and my periods stopped again. My sugar cravings turned worse and when I went to the doctor they didn't help but put me on more Prozac and anti-anxiety drugs, Concerta and now Metformin and Spironolactone and birth control. I did some research and thought I had PCOS. I got an ultrasound of my ovaries and a glucose tolerance test and it turned out I did, and was pre-diabetic.

My teeth started rotting. I needed more fillings, more crowns, and a tooth pulled. I felt dizzy often and couldn't sleep. I started cutting myself again and feeling suicidal. I ended up in the psychiatric ward again. I remember I couldn't digest food at that point – I tried eating carrots and turned orange. I didn't have a bowel movement for 17 days. I remember I told the doctors and they acted annoyed but gave me laxative after laxative and nothing worked. They sent me for an x-ray and it showed I was completely full of poop. I could barely talk at that point and they threatened me with ECT (electroconvulsive therapy). Finally they gave me some mega dose of the most vile, disgusting laxative and I was in the bathroom for two days. Horrible, but something lifted after that, and I was feeling like I could breathe again. They put me on yet another antidepressant and another anti-anxiety med and discharged me. I lost 40 lb in two months.

I was still severely depressed. I had bouts of not being able to speak and severe social anxiety. I couldn't keep anything straight but managed to try to go back to school and get a new job. I gained around 150 lb, putting my weight at around 260, in under a year. Food continued to make me itchy and anxious. My belly was constantly hurting and couldn't be touched. I craved sweets all the time and ate pints of ice cream during the night. During the day I ate bowls and bowls of cereal and boxes of crackers. I started eating meat one day out of the blue – but it still disgusted me and I had many food issues, especially touching food. I thought it would infect me. Smells of food made me itch, both on my skin and in the back of my throat. I continued to have strange rituals around food and often longed to subsist on air. My bulimia was out of control but I stopped throwing up in August 2007 out of sheer will and exhaustion.

In March of 2008, I went to the dentist and had many, many cavities. I had a jaw infection and a tooth needed to be pulled out. I had already had two pulled out in 2005; they were totally black inside. After the extractions, over the course of the year I got a throat infection and dry sockets and then that turned into a kidney infection and bacterial pneumonia. I went on rounds of antibiotics and then got thrush, a staph infection in my throat, and yeast infections. I went on anti-fungals and got UTI's. The UTI's turned into kidney infections and I got put on antibiotics again. I got bacterial pneumonia again and a skin fungus and H1N1 (a subtype of influenza virus). I stopped digesting food and starting fainting. I had four concussions and could barely breathe. I lost 150 lb in a year. I went to doctor after doctor and finally got a blood test for Celiac disease. It was positive and then I had an endoscopy. My tests showed flattened villi and GERD, so the celiac diagnosis stuck.

That was in November 2009. On the gluten-free diet alone, by March I was able to taper off all my medicine (I was on tons!). Doctors had always told me I would need to be on antidepressants my whole life or else I would have another suicide attempt. I felt so much better! Different! I remember thinking: is this how other people feel?

But my sugar cravings were still rampant. Anxiety lessened, but didn't subside completely. I ate packaged gluten-free food like there was no tomorrow! I gained back 80 lb in six months. All the GF cookies, cakes, brownies, and pasta. My stomach continued to hurt. I suddenly was unable to drink coffee – it sent me to the floor dizzy. I had been drinking pots of coffee for years since I was 10 or 11! Also, suddenly I couldn't smoke cigarettes anymore. I would get this strange feeling after smoking and feel completely drugged. I stopped one day after smoking a pack a day for 15 years. Also, the gluten-free diet was starting to make me feel bad. My joints hurt terribly, I couldn't sleep and I couldn't get up in the morning most days. And now I started having reactions to different foods. My migraines increased. 'Natural Flavors' made my face swell up, soy lecithin (and then all soy) started to give me rashes on my shins, corn and tapioca gave me rashes on my forearms, and everything gave me a stomach ache. Smells started to bother me too. All hair and bath products gave me terrible migraines. I took out dairy. Then I found a book by Sally Fallon *Nourishing Traditions* and knew it was the right path for me. I read the book obsessively and started to cut out all sugars except raw honey starting in August 2010. I tried soaking grains but found I couldn't digest them. For the first time in my life I started to come alive and learn how to cook. My body started dictating what I needed. I went to the store and suddenly bought collard greens because they looked and smelled good, even though I had no clue how to cook them! This happened with a lot of foods.

The process of nourishing myself became sacred as I tried my hand at roasting chickens, making stock weekly, making home-made soup, eating livers, and fermenting! How I loved it and how much better I felt! I lost weight naturally and everything seemed to be going well. I craved chicken skin and often wanted to eat it every day. But I continued to have new food sensitivities – eventually taking out this and that, nipping and tucking and juggling new symptoms every day.

Unfortunately, my periods stopped and I gained 60 lb from December to March 2011. I started eating 2 lb of raw honey a week by the spoon, in my sleep. All the old sugar-craving patterns returned. I found a farmer who could give me some raw milk, and that helped my brain tremendously, but not my stomach. I was bloated from the milk, but my blood sugar felt so stable! I didn't have to bring four coolers with me when I left the house. That was enough to push me towards the GAPS Diet.

I had read the *GAPS book* last August when I bought Nourishing Traditions, and I thought 'oh I don't know if I can do that...' After reading it again, the new edition, and the *GAPS Guide*, I knew it was what I needed to do.

The story of food and healing is the primary story of my life. And although I didn't always see it that way, I know now that it is a calling, and I want to help people with GAPS, food, and healing.

I started GAPS in May 2011 and have been on the Introduction Diet for six months. The GAPS Diet has totally changed my brain! I am calmer, less anxious, and able to be my real authentic self with others, without the noise that has been in my brain constantly since childhood. My depression has lifted to the point of being unnoticeable; and this is in a woman, who was told all her life that, if she went off her medicine, she would be permanently hospitalized! This is the true gift and miracle of GAPS.

It is amazing how I can handle things now! Before, even the smallest thing would send me into spirals of panic and anxiety. I can now plan and approach life as I never have before! I feel like I am part of the world. I have become much more able to speak to people and say what I mean – my social anxiety has lessened greatly. My stomach, for the first time in my life, has flattened. I used to have constant pain in my upper abdomen that has currently gone down, and when it did, my eyes became brighter and clearer, my vision improved, and my head further quieted. My skin has become softer and I hope it gets even more soft – I have had dry, rashy skin my whole life and feel it is improving from the inside out! A film I had inside my mouth and on my teeth all my life has gone, and I no longer cough up phlegm all day long. My nails are getting stronger whereas before they used to chip and split. The pain in my joints has almost completely resolved itself... and my asthma is cured! My seasonal allergies have also lifted, and my blood sugar is completely stable!! These are just the most noticeable symptoms, and I know many more will reveal themselves.

I love that GAPS allows you to truly listen and be in communication with your body. GAPS food is like a language that speaks to your body! GAPS has truly changed my life and my world view. I now understand that everything is connected to the health of your gut. I want to spread this message to others as I continue to heal. I applied for the Cooking and Culinary Traditions programme that Jessica Prentice runs at Three Stone Hearth Community Supported Kitchen in Berkeley, California, and got in. She is speaking at the WAPF conference this year, and I totally admire her vision. I want to spread the GAPS message through cooking and healing others with food, and I think that cooking at her kitchen and learning from her while continuing the GAPS Diet is a great first step. I want to be a face of GAPS in the Traditional Foods community in Berkeley at Three Stone Hearth and then bring my skill back to Minneapolis, Minnesota, in order to help people who are struggling there. I want to spread the GAPS message!! Right now I am trying to raise money to move and live there for four months, because I received a scholarship for the actual programme. I am sure I will find a way.

Dr Natasha, thank you from the bottom of my heart for creating the GAPS Diet! You have changed my life and led me to greater and greater health. It hasn't been easy, but it is a million times easier than all the pain, sickness, and suffering I have been through. I am the very PICTURE of GAPS, and I can heal. You are so wise and I feel blessed to have found the programme, thank you dear Dr Natasha!!! I will continue on my GAPS journey and if I can heal from what I used to call a lifetime of allergies, digestive stress, celiac, suicidal depression, cutting, eating disorders, hypoglycaemia, anxiety, and asthma – now I just call it GAPS – then anyone can!

A comment from Dr Natasha

What a harrowing story! Thank you so much, Lydia, for sharing it with the world! Many people don't understand what it is like to be in that situation. Your story makes the reader almost live it and feel it. God bless you for pulling yourself out of it!

12

Kathleen Bush

Key words: digestive problems, blood sugar instability, rosacea, anxiety, depression, chronic sinusitis

My story is as follows. I was a large baby: 9 lb 11 oz, born in1955. My paediatrician told my mother that since I was a large baby, she should start me on whole milk sooner rather than later. I was formula fed, of course, and started on whole milk within the first few months of my life. By the time I was two and a half, I ended up with pneumonia and a 106.6°F (41.4°C) temperature. I was rushed to the hospital, where I spent time receiving antibiotics and recovering. This was probably my first introduction to antibiotics. As you can see, between the whole milk at an extremely early age and then the antibiotic at two and a half, my poor little gut had a rough start in life.

As a child, I was plagued by chronic sore throats and ear infections. I had my tonsils out when I was seven. It was at this age that I also developed Tourette Syndrome (I was fortunate to all but outgrow it sometime in high school.) When I reached puberty, and being a typical American on a typical American diet, I began to experience anxiety, difficulty coping with stress, and blood sugar highs and lows. I was clearly dealing with GAPS.

Knowing a little about my family of origin will help round out the picture of GAPS that has been present therein my whole life. Mom had several health challenges, including two autoimmune disorders, blood clotting disorders, as well as chronic low blood pressure and severe hypothyroidism. My older sister was diagnosed with schizophrenia at the age of 14, and has never recovered; she is now 62. Other disorders that have been present for at least two, and in some cases three generations of my family of origin include: depression; anxiety; OCD,

Tourette Syndrome, processing-cognition errors; alcoholism; insomnia; social phobia; autoimmune disorders; and difficulty coping with stress.

I have always had a milk sensitivity, and have stayed away from it most of my adult life. I knew that this probably left me deficient in calcium, but I didn't feel good about taking a calcium supplement. Fortunately I have been able to tolerate cheese.

In my 40s, I developed a skin rash on my face. I went to a dermatologist, who told me it was rosacea, and prescribed a regimen of tetracycline. It definitely cleared up the rash, but I remember asking him at some point how long a person could safely stay on tetracycline. He said that I could stay on it for the rest of my life. At some point, after a year of being on the antibiotic, I took myself off it, believing that it was not normal to be on antibiotics long-term. For several years, the rash stayed at bay, but then it returned. I went to a different dermatologist, and was told the same thing, i.e. I needed to be on tetracycline. I went back on it, but this time I experimented to see how little I could take and still have clear skin. At first, I took only one capsule a week, then I cut back to one every two weeks. Once a week worked better than every two weeks, so I stayed on one capsule a week for a couple more years.

During this time, I talked with a friend of mine who told me she was sure I could find a natural cure for the 'rosacea' (which I now believe was eczema). So I began to do internet research. At the same time, another friend of mine introduced me to *Gut And Psychology Syndrome*. She had read it, and wanted to share it with me because it addresses schizophrenia, and she knows that my sister is schizophrenic.

I began to read it, hoping to be enlightened about schizophrenia, and was astounded the further I read, realizing that I was reading about my family of origin. I stayed up late two nights to finish the book. As I realized that my family of origin has had GAPS issues as long as I've been alive, so much began to make sense to me that I had never understood. Most importantly, I understood why Mom and all her daughters suffered from related disorders: we all shared the same gut flora!

I began the GAPS protocol immediately. I still remember the date: 29 March 2008. The results were immediate:

1. My blood sugar spikes and plummets disappeared overnight.
2. My blood pressure, which had always been very low but had begun to creep upward, went back down.
3. The chronic bloating I had experienced for years, particularly in my abdomen, legs and ankles, began to subside.
4. My face cleared up.
5. My ability to deal with stress began to improve.
6. My mild depression began to subside.
7. My anxiety began to subside.
8. My central stomach pain went away.
9. The pain in my left lower quadrant went away.
10. My chronic congestion went away.
11. My chronic sinus infections went away.
12. I lost 15 lb.

I am now in my third year of being on the diet. I have had many failures during this time, as I have experimented with how little sugar and white flour I can get away with. Each and every time I have come to the same conclusion: sugar and white flour need to be permanently out of my diet. Every month I am stronger than the month previous in terms of refusing to give in to my sugar and white flour addiction. My daughter, who recently started her three boys on the GAPS Diet, has been such an inspiration to me as she has rolled up her sleeves and begun to try one recipe after another. It is pure joy to have one of my children experiencing the joy of being on the GAPS Diet. My other daughter has been very receptive to the diet as well, and has made important dietary changes in her life. She's in her last year of college, and she said the thing she's looking forward to most upon graduation is having time to prepare real food again!

I have become an avid GAPS missionary ever since reading *Gut And Psychology Syndrome*. It felt right from the first reading – I've now read it seven times – and, as the proof is in the pudding, the fact that 12 troublesome aspects of my health have improved is continued evidence that the principles contained in the book are true. The GAPS Diet has revolutionized my life! I can never say enough good things about this diet. And I can never adequately thank Dr Natasha for sharing this life-saving information with the world. I believe with all my heart that this work should receive the Nobel Prize in medicine.

Recently I have experimented with juicing, and have come to be convinced of its virtue. I have been juicing for breakfast and lunch almost every day for the past five weeks. For several years, I had been experiencing intermittent side pain, which recently had become chronic. (I have researched symptoms of an ailing gall bladder, and I do have some of them.) The juicing has caused the pain to dissipate. In addition, I have lost 15 pounds and have experienced a calming effect in my entire body.

Since I began juicing at the end of May, I have finally finally overcome the sugar/carbs addiction. During the last five years, I proved to myself over and over and over that when I deviated from the diet, I experienced symptoms ranging from the above-mentioned side pain to bloating, but when I adhere to the diet, I am pain free. Bottom line: I have proved in my own body the virtue of the diet as a sustainable lifestyle, and one I will be on for the rest of my life. I have come to learn through experience that freedom from degenerative disease brought on by unhealthy life choices is a choice in and of itself. The older I get, the more I cherish my health and respect the body I was given to pass through mortality in.

Thank you, once again, Dr Natasha, for having shared with the world the life-saving knowledge you have been blessed with. My daughter is now a staunch advocate of the GAPS, and has her three small children adhering to it. She told me yesterday that she would have loved to have shared her testimonial as well, but she did not get it to you in time. She has an impressive story to tell regarding guiding her two oldest boys back to health through the diet. Both of us share our knowledge and experience whenever we have an opportunity, and have shared the GAPS book with many.

A comment from Dr Natasha

Thank you, Kathleen, for sharing your story!

It is particularly interesting to see the family background of a typical GAPS family. There are many families like this in our modern world with GAPS health problems, such as depression, schizophrenia, emotional instability, addictive personality, allergies and auto-immunity.

It is wonderful that Kathleen's daughters have become acquainted with GAPS and are implementing it in their lives and the lives of their families. Thanks to Kathleen, her branch of the family can protect their offspring from following the pattern of disease of their predecessors. As a result this branch of the family will be able to enjoy good health in their lives!

13

S.K. Smith

Key words: Depersonalisation Syndrome (DP), chronic fatigue, depression, lack of stamina, apathy, poor immunity, vegetarian, anxiety, menstrual problems

I am still in the early stages of GAPS, having started the GAPS Introduction Diet eight months ago. I am hoping for more improvements over the long term, but the results so far have been extremely encouraging. Before finding GAPS I found it almost impossible to force myself to get out of bed, or to do any physical exercise. I felt as if I was drugged – my head was 'foggy' (although I could think perfectly well). My emotional state was hard to describe, but I was very depressed and apathetic, as if I did not have the energy to care about anything, or to protest if anything went wrong. These days, I am able to run short distances, I bounce out of bed easily in the mornings, and I feel physically strong and mentally strong too. I am altogether a different person! I have become very passionate about GAPS and am always thinking about how we can make it widely known.

Here is my story: I first came to GAPS because of two particularly worrying problems, but in addition, I had various other things suggesting to me that my body was not really well as a whole.

For many years I had, with increasing severity, a condition known as Depersonalisation Syndrome (DP). This can be seen on PET scans, which show that one area of the brain is inactive. The experience of DP for me is that I do not feel awake, but as if I am dreaming, and I have the sense that my brain is not properly comprehending my surroundings, even though I am able to be factually accurate about everything, and to respond to my surroundings in ways that other people find appropriate. Relationships are difficult, since the emotional meaning of situations is difficult to interpret. People and places seem unfamiliar, and I cannot remember how things used to feel when I was well. I don't feel the normal range of emotions, and often feel emotions happening in my body without me connecting to them, as if I am a robot. This experience is frightening and bewildering.

More recently I had also developed fatigue. I had become lethargic and apathetic, quite unlike my usual self. Normally I would be very active – instead I only wanted to be allowed to stay in bed, and forcing myself into activity would only increase this feeling. If I caught a cold or stomach bug, it would go on for a long time, and then I would be under par for many weeks.

I decided to try GAPS after reading the book, even though I was not under the supervision of a doctor or naturopath. I began with Full GAPS Diet, as an experiment, to see how I would feel after a short time. Within three days I was feeling so different that I became more confident that it was the right approach for me. Before GAPS I had begun to take for granted my feelings of 'foggy headedness' and the sense of every small task being a struggle to get my brain to focus properly. Inside, I had no trouble focusing – I could write and speak clearly – but my surroundings seemed to be hazy and hard to grasp, and I found it hard to respond to them, even though to others I appeared normal. I have never read anywhere a description of this sensation, yet it was very powerful for me, and made my life difficult as well as distressing. With every day that I was on GAPS I felt this sensation lessening, and was able to be more effective in my work.

Coming from a vegetarian wholefood diet, it was a difficult transition to make to the GAPS Introduction Diet. So I decided to wean myself off GAPS illegal foods slowly, and in the meantime to try to nourish myself with lots of fat, as well as plenty of vegetables and fermented foods. After six months I had managed to come to terms with eating without dairy, fruit, beans or nuts, and went into the Introduction Diet. During the preparation time I had already started becoming stronger physically. Instead of staying in bed until 10 or 11 a.m. unable to get up, I could get up at 7 a.m. regularly and not need to sleep again during the day. I began to feel more alive, and more connected to other people, which to a person with DP means a great deal. I also noticed my appetite changing. I no longer craved sweet things, but wanted to eat a lot of meat and fish.

However, it was important for me to do the Introduction Diet, I felt, because I was still unable to do normal things like housework or the lightest form of exercise, and also because I was hopeful that the DP would improve. I found Intro very difficult in the beginning. It seemed to release a tide of emotions, and made me feel ill. I was unable to eat much fat, as it would simply make me nauseous, and I felt terribly hungry. Experimenting with broth making was challenging too, as I battled with feelings of revulsion towards some meat I tried. I tried one sip of coconut kefir and it triggered a headache which lasted for two days.

Nevertheless, over the next three months I noticed some changes:

- losing weight steadily (I had been overweight);
- a lovely feeling in my stomach after eating, instead of the dull pain I had taken for granted;
- an awakening of my taste buds so that food tasted the way it had done when I was a child;
- a heightened sensitivity to smell, making certain chemical smells very offensive;
- the thumb that always hurt stopped hurting;
- my periods, which had been irregular and painful became regular and pain-free;
- my anxiety levels reduced dramatically, and my mood was immeasurably more optimistic;
- losing strength to the point where it was overwhelmingly exhausting to even go upstairs;
- feeling connected to other people again, and able to remember more of my life prior to DP;
- *not* feeling deprived, as I had expected, but grateful for how satisfying I suddenly found food to be, and astonished at the depletion I must have been suffering for so long.

The GAPS Intro Diet was a kind of crisis, as I struggled to learn this new way of shopping, cooking and eating. I decided I was willing to go through all the feelings of hunger and weakness because I wanted so badly to get well. I knew, since I had felt so different on the Full GAPS Diet, that many of the horrid sensations I was experiencing were because I was detoxifying. Though they were so unpleasant, I felt glad to know that the toxins were coming out of my body and would leave me generally healthier.

There was an unexpected part of this new phase of my life. I had previously shopped at supermarkets. Now I was visiting my local farmers' market every weekend, and shopping at local Turkish supermarkets, fishmongers and butcher's during the week. The experience of shopping in this way was very different, because I felt a connection both to the people who were serving me, and to the food. I was being served by the people who collected the meat from the farms, or placed the orders from the farmers in Turkey, or even by the farmers themselves. They recognised me and were friendly to me, and I started to feel that I was part of a community. I might not have meant much to them personally, but I was contributing to their environment by bringing them my money and my appreciation. I began to have a tangible feeling of how much they were contributing to mine by selling me the food that was making me well. This sense of our interdependence seemed to create a particular atmosphere.

My kitchen started to look more homely, too. Suddenly there were jars of fermenting things all over the place, and my fridge was always full of lovely looking vegetables. The smell of broth permeated the house.

Eventually a breakthrough came. I found I had much more energy, and saw this increasing weekly. I felt a sudden difference in my frame of mind as well. I felt angry and impatient, where before I had felt passive and resigned. It was as if I suddenly had enough strength to care about how I was feeling. My immune system seemed to wake up, too. Suddenly I was allergic to everything. My periods also stopped again. I was confused by the mixture of improvement and negative things, and also desperately hungry. I continued to add in more foods, which did help the hunger.

Since that time, I have seen steady improvement in all the physical aspects of my fatigue to the point where I could begin to exercise again. I began to try other things to aid my healing, and saw enormous benefits from doing the liver flush, colon cleansing, and from having treatment for periodontal disease. I also acquired an Earthing sheet, which may have helped, and definitely gave me better sleep and general wellbeing.

This month I have returned again to the GAPS Introduction Diet – this time with no symptoms of die-off or detox. In fact, I have felt much better than since before I started the diet at all. I am intending to re-introduce foods more slowly this time. Interestingly, on the second day of this Intro, I had a period – my first in five months.

To date, not every one of my problems has been resolved, but I can run, dance, do decorating, go for long walks, and carry heavy loads – without tiring. This is a far cry from when a trip to the local shop seemed like a marathon, and exercise was unthinkable. However, my GAPS journey has felt like more than just a journey from illness to health. It has felt like a journey from death to life! I don't like to dwell on how I felt this time a year ago. The way I feel now is another world, where I feel properly alive, and vibrating with it. I also feel more connected to love, and much more able to share love with others. That has meant as much to me as having my bodily functions restored, and I am grateful for it with all my heart. This feels like a SECRET which, if only people knew how it feels, would be valued the world over!

A comment from Dr Natasha

This story shows how very individual and unique everybody's experience is. S.K. Smith had to go through ups and downs several times in these short eight months. It is a credit to her that she did not get discouraged and persevered with the GAPS Programme, coming back to the Introduction Diet more than once. Every time her symptoms were becoming milder and she derived more and more benefit. Another lesson to learn from S.K. Smith is that she listened to her body and took things slowly. Being kind to yourself, and taking things at the pace which your body can cope with, is very important and can make all the difference. Thank you very much for your story!

14

Anonymous

Key word: depression

Five years ago I moved away from an area that I had lived in most of my life, approximately 45 years. I came to a new area where I knew very few people. I left my adult son behind and my lovely home and all my friends. I was lonely and in shock. I fell into a deep depression; I had to be hospitalized twice. When I got out of the hospital my psychiatrist put me on Lexapro and Abilify. I slowly improved, but the drugs helped me gain 50 lb. Now I feared the possibility of diabetes.

Fortunately, I found a wonderful GAPS practitioner who helped me get back on track. I AM NO LONGER DEPRESSED! I FEEL WONDERFUL AND I AM LOSING WEIGHT FOR THE FIRST TIME IN YEARS! Thank heaven I was able to find help, and I hope my letter will help someone else! I hope to be totally free of antidepressants soon with the help of my GAPS practitioner.

A comment from Dr Natasha

Thank you very much for your letter!

The human brain is a very hungry organ, it needs feeding all the time, and the best foods for it come from animal products: meat, meat stock and bone broth, animal fats, fresh eggs, fresh fish and fermented high-fat dairy. Standard Western diet does not provide good nutrition for the brain, and when it is starving it cannot function too well. Periods of stress drain nutrients out of the body at an alarming rate, so it is very easy to run out of them and put your brain into starvation. And if on top of that your digestive system is not functioning well, then depression, anxiety or any other 'mental' disorder is just around the corner.

15

R. Fiano

Key words: psoriasis, psoriatic arthritis

I have suffered from psoriasis for more than a decade. At first it was localised. It appeared on my chest, back and scalp. Nothing I was worried about until the company I worked with underwent major restructuring in 2010. The uncertainty and stress affected my health to the point that I developed psoriatic arthritis in January 2011. I was made redundant and started to treat my condition with my mainstream doctor. However, my condition was not improving noticeably. So with my doctor's blessing, I asked to increase my dosage (Methotraxate and folic acid), but my pharmacist took me aside to find out if I was closely monitored. It became clear to me that my treatment was not as safe as I thought. I decided to go the nutrition route. I cut out acidic fruits, cheese, processed sugar, ate more organic foods, honey, cider vinegar and reduced my salt intake. My doctor was furious that I stopped the medication without her consent, but slowly my joint pains disappeared, and I had renewed faith in my long-held (but forgotten) belief that our body can heal itself if only we give it the right weapons.

Unfortunately, the psoriasis part of my condition flared up in August 2011 until it covered my entire body. Once again, I reverted to mainstream medicine and was of course disappointed.

Then I attended a lecture by Dr Campbell-Bride on 25 March 2012. In five minutes she gave me the insights I needed to recover:

1. My skin type requires twice the normal sun exposure to produce vitamin D, which helps ANY health problem.
2. Psoriasis is a case of self-immunity: I needed to change my diet and use probiotics to regain that balance.

3   The condition gradually built up over a decade at least before
    spreading the year before. Therefore it was improbable that I would
    be rid of it overnight. Patience would be needed.
4   A rule of thumb for all skin products: ultimately, if I can't put it in
    (eating it), I shouldn't put it on (apply it to my skin – 'eating' it
    through my skin).

Following a few tips from her book *Gut And Psychology Syndrome*, in
April 2012 I started using olive oil on my skin. I cooked vegetable
stews, added Neways Advanced Probiotic to my diet (1 capsule a day at
first, then gradually increased until I had 3 a day), cod liver oil and
fish, and I banned pasta and rice. I started bathing in organic oats
instead of commercial bath salts, I also had a few phototherapy
sessions, which my mainstream doctor thought were the ultimate solution, but I had a few reactions to those too. I endured the probiotic die-
off reactions for a few weeks, then by May 2012 my skin had cleared!
At the time of writing this, June 2012, my skin looks better than it has
ever been. In the process, I have lost a stone. I am now my ideal
weight, I feel healthy and look healthy again!

What we call progress – modern civilisation – is little more than
junk packaged in glittery glamorous stuff. There has been a worldwide
propaganda that is killing all of us slowly.

I thought cholesterol was all bad. WRONG! We need cholesterol to
process vitamins, it is a PR stunt from the food industry to encourage
eating processed stuff that they market rather than natural organic stuff.

I thought animal fat was bad. WRONG! Scientists know that it is not
the principal cause of fattening. Who benefits from us believing that?
The food industry.

Sun exposure gives cancer. WRONG! Too much of a good thing is
indeed bad, but sun exposure helps the body create vitamin D.
Processed foods have next to no nutritional value and are much more
dangerous. It's been scientifically proven.

The 'science' stuff that gets through to the general public is mainly
the stuff that is endorsed by a wealthy organisation. The aim is the
same as usual: MORE PROFIT.

I took a holistic approach to my illness. The right combination of
diet, probiotics, vitamins and minerals, change of lifestyle (reduce

stress by doing more of what I love doing) and letting go of the belief that mainstream (medicine or food or products) must be the best way. Just because the mainstream view was that the Earth was flat did not make it correct. I am glad that there are doctors out there, like Dr Campbell-McBride, prepared to challenge incorrect mainstream views. Thanks a million for your invaluable insights that gave me my life back!

I have documented my journey on my blog (link below) http://www.fourthreethings.com/things/view/11ninefourninetwofive/do-something-about-my-psoriasis

A comment from Dr Natasha

Thank you for this wonderful story! Psoriasis is becoming more and more common, and many sufferers are led to believe that it is incurable. This story demonstrates that there is a way of removing psoriasis from your life, and removing it permanently!

16

Starlene D. Stewart

Key words: depression, painful feet / plantar fasciitis, back pain, arthritis, anxiety, asthma, allergies, PMS, blood sugar instability, fatigue, mood instability, overweight

I am a 47-year-old woman who has had great success on GAPS. I had sworn off dieting 16 years ago, and I only decided to give GAPS a chance because my husband had been diagnosed with ulcerative colitis. While reading *Gut and Psychology Syndrome* I became interested to find out whether my depression and fatigue could be addressed. That was all I really hoped to get from GAPS. My husband started out with me on GAPS but he found the diet too daunting. He did learn what was causing most of his problems and has eliminated certain foods, and I still hope that he will eventually join me for complete healing of his disease.

I started on GAPS in December 2009 and have been chronicling my progress at my blog GAPS Diet Journey (http://www.gapsdietjourney.com). Within two weeks of starting on the Full GAPS I was delighted and amazed to realize that my two painful conditions had completely ceased: my feet stopped hurting and my back stopped stiffening while sleeping. This healing caused me to rejoice and fully commit to the healing protocol.

My feet were very painful and it was difficult for me to stand for any length of time. I'd found a brand of men's casual wear shoes that had a thick cushion, which eased the pain, and I had to wear them every waking moment. I had been diagnosed with plantar fasciitis a year or so earlier and it hurt to stand in the shower barefoot. I had to put shoes on just to go from my bed to the bathroom in the middle of the night. However, almost like magic on Day 13 of doing Full GAPS, my feet stopped hurting. I have actually been able to enjoy wearing fashion-able shoes!

Also within that time I realized that my back had stopped stiffening up during the night. Ever since a serious bout with pneumonia in 2002 when I was sicker than I'd ever been in my entire life and had been bedridden for an entire month, I found I was unable to sleep longer than seven hours without my back stiffening into knots and hurting so badly that I had no choice but to get out of bed. Even then it took an hour or two to relax, unkink and completely stop hurting. This, I believe, caused me to be quite sleep-deprived since I work outside of the home and could only nap on the weekends. It was like a miracle to be able to actually sleep for longer periods of time! I feel that sleep is vitally important to healing; now I can sleep for nine or more hours and my back doesn't hurt at all.

At my blog I posted a six-month update and listed all the healing I'd experienced. I was sleeping better, the brain fog had cleared, I was no longer 'losing words' (I'd be speaking and couldn't think of the word I was looking for), I found I was able to concentrate better, the mild depression had lifted (before GAPS I'd been taking kava kava, some-times daily for anxiety and that had disappeared), I was no longer crying about every little thing, my wrists stopped hurting, I was no longer dropping things, my strength and stamina were better, I had more energy, I actually wanted to spend time with my husband again, I was no longer feeling fatigued, my appetite had decreased, I was no longer overeating, skin tags were disappearing from my body, I was no longer having mild road rage, no longer having constipation (an occa-sional problem pre-GAPS), my stomach was no longer bloated, my ankles and fingers had not swelled up since I'd been on GAPS (an occa-sional problem pre-GAPS), I was no longer having blood sugar drops where I'd get nervous and shaky from not eating right away, my lower back used to ache when I washed dishes and that stopped.

The most significant healing at nine months into my GAPS jour-ney was being able to go off my asthma medication! I had been taking a corticosteroid *flovent* for eight years since the pneumonia in 2002. I was taking the lowest dose of *flovent* (40mcg), two puffs once daily. I tried to get off it at about three months into GAPS, but that was too soon. I went back on it for a few months and then slowly began tapering down and finally took my last dosage at the end of August 2010. I have also had one cold since that time, had only slight breathing problems (a cold can really exacerbate asthma) and used my *albuterol* twice on the worst day. Other than that, I had no breathing problems. I've also noticed that my allergies seem to be non-existent. I used to sneeze a lot and my sinuses were constantly swollen.

At one year I shared that I had increased energy, my blood sugar had stabilized so well that I could now eat only three meals a day without snacks in between! No more PMS and pain-free periods! I am no longer fatigued like I was for years before starting GAPS. I am no longer having anxiety attacks and crying frequently and hating my life.

Finally, I have lost 70 lb almost effortlessly. For years I swore I loved carbs more than my own mother, and could never, ever give them up. Just the thought of giving them up would start giving me cravings and I would end up binging. But getting off carbohydrates allowed me to stop the addiction to them and it has been easier than I ever imagined staying on GAPS. I did not start on GAPS to lose weight, although at 5'4" and over 232 lb, it was certainly something I could stand to do. I am still looking forward to having more energy and losing more weight and hope to see those improvements in the coming months.

One more thing you should know. I am unable to afford to eat only organic vegetables and grass-fed and organic meats. I do try to have these foods when I can afford them, but for the most part the healing I have experienced has come from eating conventionally grown foods. I do have a garden and I am able to produce some good vegetables for myself at some months of the year, so I am grateful for that. We also owned dairy goats but were unable to afford keeping them. I had tried to re-introduce dairy in March 2010, but my asthma was affected, so I decided to stay off dairy until sometime in the future. When I was able to go off my asthma medication I decided to stay off dairy products (except I am okay with ghee and butter) for one year. September 2011 will be my one year anniversary off the asthma medication and I plan to try to introduce fermented dairy and see how that goes. I have great hopes that I will be able to tolerate yogurt and kefir and aged cheese.

I heard Dr Natasha say on a podcast that she keeps her family on GAPS to prevent common maladies; I do not foresee returning to eating processed foods either as I believe most of my symptoms would return, and I was a very unhappy person prior to GAPS.

My life is so much different now, and I look forward to more healing. I thank Dr Natasha for coming up with this nutrition protocol and I thank God that I stopped being stubborn and decided to try GAPS to heal my body!

A comment from Dr Natasha

Thank you very much for your story, Starlene!

There are millions of people in the world who are struggling with the same health problems and believe that there is nothing they can do. Your experience will help them to see a way out.

Your point about food supply is very important: many people have no access to or cannot afford organic, grass-fed and pastured foods. Of course it is better to look for the best-quality foods, but many people, just like you, manage to do the programme with conventional foods and get good results.

17

Gawain Hammond

Key words: peripheral neuropathy, diarrhoea, IBS, fatigue, depression

It all started about four years ago. I was a healthy 30-year-old with a good life, I was fit and enjoyed activities like Capoeira. Initially I felt mild weakness in my muscles and felt my wit was diminished, then diarrhoea developed, and a month later I developed very intense peripheral neuropathy (PN) with intermittent fever-like symptoms. I couldn't sleep, and it felt like being swarmed by bees that were stinging constantly. I went to hospital that night and they sent me back home, as there was nothing they could do. The next day I saw my GP who diagnosed me with alcoholic neuropathy (symptoms initially begun after drinking alcohol). I abstained and was given a course of Thiamine, which after about a week did improve my symptoms dramatically. The PN symptoms gradually improved over the next 12 months, and I begun to feel a lot less anxious, but over time new symptoms began to appear and the diarrhoea persisted continually. I always felt the symptoms were linked and begun to anecdotally notice that sugar would make the peripheral neuropathy a little worse. But I was told by a doctor it was probably coincidence and that I just had IBS from stress.

Then, one day, about 18 months ago the peripheral neuropathy symptoms came back intensely. I wracked my brains as to what it could be. I didn't drink any more alcohol, I was taking 150mg of thiamine each day, so what could it be? And I suddenly realized: I had got back in to the gym and had been consuming daily protein powders full of 'complex carbs' that were basically sugar. I returned to my doctor and we thought maybe it was diabetes. But after tests I found out I definitely wasn't diabetic. Over the next two years I began to experience worsening and new symptoms: fatigue, foggy confusion, very sore joints, sleep apnea, feeling like I was getting massive electric shocks just as I dropped off to sleep, extreme sensitivity to noise, dizziness, inability to remember cash at cash machines or what people had said a few minutes before, falling asleep in the day totally exhausted. I thought I was potentially very ill, no one had any idea what was wrong with me, and no one could even understand what it felt like. Most people wrote me off as a hypochondriac. I felt very, very alone and slowly slipped into depression.

So now I knew to stay away from sugar and the PN symptoms would remain manageable. It was an improvement, so I next focused on the diarrhoea symptoms, which I felt must be connected in some way. Then one day, while trying to choose a book on IBS, I found the light! A reviewer had said that IBS books were mostly a waste of time and any potential buyer should try the GAPS Diet instead. I noted down the name of the diet and moved on.

As soon as I started reading the GAPS book I felt a weight lift off me and I felt very confident. I had finally found the cause of all my symptoms. Nothing had ever explained all my seemingly disparate symptoms any better than the GAPS. I knew at once this had a very high chance of success. So about six weeks ago I embarked on the diet.

Within these last six weeks my diarrhoea has dramatically improved, fatigue has also improved dramatically and they remain the only mild symptoms left. I have now stopped taking thiamine, which would usually make the PN symptoms return within a couple of weeks, and so far I'm feeling only mild pins and needles. I can't believe that after four years I have finally solved these health problems and I can honestly say I owe my life to this diet, as there were times when I felt the poor quality of life made me feel that I didn't want to carry on much longer living this way and living in fear of what symptoms I would get next.

In hindsight, after reading the GAPS book, I believe it's all rooted in the course of antibiotic oxytetracycline I was given for (mild) acne in my youth about 15 years ago. I was too young to know then what effects it might have, but I would never take such a long course of antibiotics now!

Many thanks for all your work! I am now getting on with life again.

A comment from Dr Natasha

Thank you for your wonderful story, Gawain! There are many forms of neuropathy and many of them are considered 'incurable'. This story has demonstrated again that all diseases begin in the gut, just as Hippocrates stated thousands of years ago! An abnormal gut flora floods the body with a river of toxicity, which can poison the nervous system and cause pathology in any part of it. As you focus on healing your gut, that flow of toxins stops, and all sorts of health problems disappear, no matter how far away from the digestive system they may be (including neuropathy).

18

Emily Jane Williams

Key words: plantar fasciitis, progressive peripheral neuropathy, eye problems

I suffered with 'plantar fasciitis' for five years, then peripheral neuropathy for the past year and a half. My plantar fasciitis, and later, progressive PN (peripheral neuropathy) had caused me huge medical bills and costs for assistance with daily needs. I expected life to be not-worth-living within a few months due to the pain and pins-and-needles sensations from my feet to my waist, from my hands to my shoulder joints, and across my back.

I started the GAPS Diet gradually: first I omitted sugar, which took only two weeks, then grains, which took five weeks, then decaf coffee (I was drinking only one mug a day), which took six weeks. I suffered severe die-off with each of those steps. I then went on the Full GAPS Diet, knowing I wouldn't be able to live through an immediate transition into the Intro Diet.

My PN pain and other symptoms reduced 95% over six weeks, so I slowly decreased my medication (Lyrica). I was taking only 25 mg at night, but spent seven weeks coming off it. I took my last dose the night before last.

I now can stand and walk as much as I need to do my daily activities. I can again press my foot on the gas and brake pedals of my car for as long as I need, so I can drive anywhere. I have a brief resurgence of mild symptoms during awakening in the morning and a bit when I stand for too long (over 10 minutes in one position). And I haven't even done GAPS properly yet! Imagine what I will feel like when I commit to the whole programme!

Although no medical doctor has determined a cause for my plantar fasciitis or my PN, I personally believe Wellbutrin (an antidepressant)

caused the plantar fasciitis that developed into PN. My symptoms began two weeks after beginning to take the Wellbutrin. The Wellbutrin also caused dramatic heart arrhythmia after taking it for three years. I quickly weaned myself off this drug and the symptoms have vanished permanently. I was taking 1/8 of a minimum dose, and the arrhythmia started immediately after I increased the dose to 3/8 of minimum.

I do not know whether I am enjoying a temporary remission or whether I have found the solution to my problem, but I believe the latter. I am so excited with my renewed health that I am heading to Costa Rica in two weeks to enjoy one week of family camp on the organic farm run by the W.A.P.F. chapter leader for Costa Rica. I'll be gone 23 July – 14 August, enough time to travel to other areas of the country before returning.

In addition to the decrease in my neuropathy symptoms, my eyesight has improved! I didn't believe it at first, but I definitely can see better at night, and the bright headlights – even the blue ones – don't hurt my eyes the way they used to for the past 15+ years! I have glaucoma and two of the three types of cataracts.

I am forever indebted to my W.A.P.F. chapter leader Carol Albrecht for telling me about Dr Natasha Campbell-McBride and the GAPS Programme. Dr Natasha's research and educational efforts have truly saved my life!

A comment from Dr Natasha

Thank you for your story, Emily Jane! Many drugs can cause neurological problems, so you may be right about the cause of your neuropathy. GAPS Diet is very dense in nutrients; it removes nutritional deficiencies quite quickly. Our nervous system is a very hungry organ, it needs feeding all the time with high-quality nutrients. On top of that, GAPS Programme restores your detoxification system, so your body starts removing toxic substances, such as drugs, very efficiently, before they can cause trouble.

19

Sherry Miller

Key words: menopause, mitral valve prolapse (MVP), anxiety

At age 30, I woke up one night with my heart racing. My husband brought me to the hospital and I was diagnosed as having MVP, mitral valve prolapse. This is a very common diagnosis in women. I was immediately put on a beta blocker and valium. This was in the late 70's. I was very active at that time and was raising two small children. I felt like the drugs were making me feel bad, so I took myself off them and then returned to the doctor. He said if I took my blood pressure regularly and felt ok, then perhaps I didn't need to take the drug at this time.

I am now 63 and have never taken any medication for this diagnosis. However, about eight years ago, well into menopause, I once again started having these rapid heart-beating episodes in the middle of the night. I would wake up out of a deep sleep with my heart racing, like I was running a marathon. It was very upsetting. You would immediately feel like it was life threatening. On two different occasions, I went to the hospital to be checked out. Both times, they insisted I was just fine and nothing was wrong with me. Of course I knew better, because these instances would happen again! I tried everything natural that I could find. Thank God for Classical 5 Element Acupuncture, which most of the time helped tremendously! I also took supplements from Standard Process along with yoga, deep breathing techniques and other therapies. Since menopause I have had more than my share of anxiety and anxiety attacks. One moment I would be fine, the next I would be a basket case for no apparent reason.

During these years, my husband and I ate very 'healthy', we thought! We ate lots of fruits, vegetables, range chicken and wild caught fish. However we ate very little animal fat and no red meat. In

February of 2010, we were told about WAPF so we joined. We ordered the *Nourishing Traditions* cookbook, *Eat Fat Lose Fat, Gut And Psychology Syndrome* and *Put Your Heart In Your Mouth!* Oh, my gosh, did our lives start to drastically change! We went from eating very little fat and no red meat to lots of fats, adding red meats and organ meats as well. We hadn't eaten red meat in over 15 years, but thought, why not? We are just not feeling as healthy as we should, and I was still having attacks in the middle of the night, along with anxiety.

We started eating lots of animal fat, and I want everyone to know that my attacks of heart racing in the middle of the night, or any other time, have vanished! My anxiety level is lower than I can ever remember and constantly improving. I had also noticed, during the same time when I was having these attacks, that my husband's heart seemed to be beating hard. When I would lie next to him, I could feel its intensity. Now, when I lie next to him, I notice a much softer, lighter beating of his heart. I am sure this is all due to the adding of animal fat, saturated fat, to our diet. Obviously our hearts needed animal fat as well as the rest of our body. Thank God for Dr Campbell-McBride's book, *Put Your Heart In Your Mouth*. I read it shortly after we joined WAPF and it convinced me we were doing the right thing!

We are constantly seeing improvements in our overall health. Over the years I have tried many new and different ways of eating; vegetarian, proper combining, metabolic typing, diet according to your blood type and more recently, only sprouted grains and flours (*Creating Heaven Through Your Plate*). None, I repeat, none of these ways of eating improved our health like eating traditional foods. One more note: we stayed on the prior ways of eating, each of them, at least one year...so we didn't jump from one to another. We gave them all adequate time to improve our health.

Conventional medicine wants to put most menopausal women on antidepressants and other drugs. Don't give in! It is not the answer. The food you eat and how you prepare it is the key to your good health. I am so glad I persisted with my search for natural means, and so grateful for dedicated women like Sally Fallon and Dr Campbell-McBride, who are truly here to help us as we aspire to become healthy individuals.

After going to the WAPF Convention and hearing Dr Campbell-McBride speak, and many others, we came home and started the GAPS Diet immediately. We have even attempted the Intro GAPS. I feel like we have a new lease on life, and control of our health. My husband and I both always believed that God perfected our bodies, so they could heal themselves if given the right tools. I spent lots of time during those 10 years searching for those tools, trying new modalities, eating the latest health diet, seeing natural practitioners in other states. I feel like we are finally HOME! Dr Campbell-McBride and Sally Fallon have given us the tools we need to be well. What we do with them is our responsibility.

My husband and I have made a commitment to teach, teach, teach and share all this incredible information. We have also opened a WAPF Chapter in our city, Lafayette, LA. We are so grateful to Dr Price and all the other scientists, doctors, practitioners and lay people who have written the books and done the research for us! It is not a new diet, but eating the traditional way – God's original plan.

A comment from Dr Natasha

Thank you, Sherry, for your story! The world is full of nutritional misinformation and it is easy to get lost in it. So many people believe the popular media and attempt various changes in their diet, thinking that this way they take good care of their health. Eating low-fat and avoiding meats, red meats in particular, is one of the most pervasive recommendations in the mainstream, and one of the most damaging. Sherry and her husband found the real information and as a result regained their good health.

20

Catherine Cruchon

Patient of Mrs Kruger-Fantoli, French-speaking Certified GAPS
Practitioner in Switzerland
Translated from French (the French text follows)

Key words: Chronic Fatigue Syndrome, reflux, dyslexia, asthma,
headaches, sleeping problems, digestive problems, candida, addiction to
grains and sugar, amenorrhea, hyperactivity, restless legs, heartburn

My name is Catherine Cruchon, I am 24 years old. Here is the story of
how I moved from being an elite sportswoman to becoming bedridden; and then getting my life back, thanks to the GAPS Programme.

First of all a little about my personality: I had always been a perfec-
tionist and a bit hyperactive. I try to be the best in all that I undertake.
For example, I never get involved in anything I am not good at,
because I do not like to be behind. All my life I had a lot of energy and
a very busy schedule: gymnastics, music, running, and then from 13
years of age three sessions of rowing a week.

I was seldom ill, and despite being a daredevil and a tomboy I had
never broken any bones. I trusted my body and felt invincible. However,
thinking back, the first symptoms were already present. Any whiff of hot
season would give me headaches. My body managed the changes of
temperature badly: I always felt too warm. I was not therefore a
supporter of sunbathing; I almost never tanned and remained 'white'.

I did not sleep well either: I would wake up two or three times per
night. I remember thinking that it was simply necessary for me to exercise vigorously enough every day to succeed in falling asleep.

Then I was diagnosed as dyslexic with extreme delays in reading; so
I had to have special lessons for a year and a half. At the same time, I
developed asthma and was put on Ventolin and Cortisone.

During adolescence I tried cannabis, but it did not agree with me. Just two inhalations of the smoke gave me a 'bad trip': I lost any sense of reality and felt that my personality got split in two. This feeling of loss of control scared me enough to make me stop the cigarettes and cannabis for good.

Despite all that, I had a good childhood: school was easy, I played a lot of sport and managed well. I had some problems in making friends, but apart from that I could not complain. My hyperactive behaviour has never bothered me; on the contrary I was proud to succeed in so many things as well as doing my studies. I had energy and motivation all day long and I loved it!

In my twenties I became a member of the Swiss national rowing team. My life was filled by intensive training and I also had a job as a winegrower. I had 11 sessions of training a week, plus regular training camps. And when I had a chance I would go out with my friends. I felt strong and happy: brilliant friends, exciting job, and training for the rowing championships.

It was in my twenties however that I started becoming lethargic and tired all the time. At first I was too tired to walk after training, then too tired to dress up after training. I had no more energy to answer the telephone at the end of the day, and my results in training became poor. I then began having pain in my limbs which was hard to define, something inside between the muscle and the bone, as if my nerves were compressed. Finally I felt so much pain in my legs and feet that I could not walk anymore. I felt like I was carrying 300 kg all the time, while my legs were replaced by painful pieces of wood.

At the same time I developed fermentation in my stomach, which made eating uncomfortable and affected my sleep. I felt ravenously hungry regularly, with cold sweats and a feeling of weakness, despite having a full stomach. I could not digest many foods, especially raw vegetables, food sat like a stone in my stomach. Often during meals my tummy would feel so uncomfortable that I had to lie down.

I lost a lot of hair and it became very fine. I became even more sensitive to warm weather, sweating profusely. But the most difficult thing to cope with was severe fatigue. It was more a lack of energy and a feeling of weakness, than a need to sleep. I had no energy to do anything despite having slept for 12 hours at night. At first the tiredness was cyclical, for two to three weeks I would be full of energy. Then, for an identical time, I slept continuously. But at the end the fatigue had become permanent.

My burning stomach (which often felt like hunger) would occupy my thoughts to the point that I couldn't do anything but eat. I became addicted to bread and more bread and other starches. I was like a drug addict and only bread could reduce the feeling of hunger. I could eat 300g of bread every few hours: I ate in the morning, at midday, at 6 p.m., at 9 p.m., at midnight and I had to get up again at about 4 a.m. to eat more; without it I could not sleep. And at every meal I had to have a minimum of 150g of bread or some sweet grain. It had become unthinkable to eat vegetables or fruit. I could not drink water because it aggravated my heartburn. I ate lots of dairy products and sugar (I consumed 3 kg of chocolate spread in 1 month). I ate constantly to reduce the burning in my stomach. I had lost the feeling of satiety. Luckily for me, I do not put weight on easily; the number of calories I was consuming was frightening!

Paradoxically, it took me a while to realize that these symptoms were not normal. It's as if I erased this data in my head to be able to continue with my lifestyle. I told my doctor about my fatigue, but all the usual tests came back normal. As my doctor did not get worried, I persuaded myself that this problem was only temporary. There was a suspicion of infectious mononucleosis, but it turned out to be false and could not explain my symptoms. The same story with my menstruations: they stopped three years ago. Yet, all my hormonal tests were normal. My gynaecologist could not explain it and prescribed the pill to trigger my periods ...

Finally, I was so debilitated that I could not calculate 2+2, my brain was completely out of order. It was impossible for me to organize anything or plan for the future. Sometimes I felt like banging my head on the wall. Honestly I was afraid to be hospitalized into a psychiatric facility, if I told anyone about how I felt. I could now understand what autistic children feel like; if I was a child I probably would have become autistic.

I got seriously worried. I had no energy left to go out, to study or work. It was very sad. I had no recognizable illness, yet I was very ill and unable to do anything. I worried that my doctor might diagnose me with depression and declare it a cause of my disability. I understood that when doctors don't know what's wrong with you they usually prescribe antidepressants. I was not prepared to go that way. As a sportswoman I was used to pushing my body beyond limits; I wanted to be in control without my brain dulled by antidepressants on top of all the confusion I already had. I was already taking several drugs without any effect: a drug for heartburn, Ritalin for hyperactivity and a drug for the restless legs. The more doctors you go to the more drugs you are prescribed: all to reduce symptoms and none to deal with the cause of the problem. At age 24 I was given all these drugs to be taken indefinitely.

I friend told me about GAPS a while ago. At the time I didn't look at it seriously, but now I was prepared to do anything. So, one Sunday I stopped all medication and started the GAPS Diet. Only a day later I woke up so different that at first I did not believe it myself. I still had the heartburn, as well as several other things, but I was full of energy! I remember running up the stairs skipping two steps at a time, having quick movements and a smile from ear to ear. At that point I felt like I had come alive again! I then made an appointment to see Mrs Kruger-Fantoli (French-speaking Certified GAPS Practitioner in Switzerland) to get proper guidance on how to implement the GAPS Programme.

The first brilliant thing was that I finally had an explanation for my illness: I finally understood where it came from! It all started from avoiding the sun. And my hair thinning, and fatigue and my digestive symptoms – it all suddenly became logical.

The GAPS Programme was not easy as I was just starting at the university of Oregon. Here I was, studying wine-making at university, and I could not drink wine or any other alcohol! I could not taste any of the good dishes my fellow students were making or go to any of the succulent restaurants of Portland. Furthermore it is much more difficult to make acquaintance with people if you cannot share a drink, food or even coffee with them! On top of that it takes a lot of organization to obtain all the food necessary and planning to have always a ready meal and a filled fridge.

I confess not to have been very strict at my arrival in Oregon: new skylines, new friends, weekend camping, BBQs, drink, coffee, holidays... But in less than two weeks I was back in bed with severe fatigue... I went back on the strict GAPS Introduction Diet and as if by magic my energy returned. Yes, it is not easy not to be able to share meals and drink with people. But I remember how I felt when I broke the diet, and it becomes well worthwhile to stick to it.

I hope that one day GAPS will become so well known, that there will be restaurants and cafes serving GAPS food and drink. A large number of people have questioned me about GAPS and came to the conclusion that they too have it. I am convinced that a good proportion of people on this planet will not be able to continue eating the standard Western food much longer without having more and more health problems – problems for which classical medicine has nothing to offer.

To finish, I would like to say a huge thank you to Dr N Campbell-McBride for her research and work. I would like to thank Mrs Krüger-Fantoli for her guidance and recommendations, my parents and my sisters for their help and their support, and my friends for their understanding! Without you I would not have been here!

Thank you from the bottom of my heart!

A comment from Dr Natasha

Thank you for your story, Catherine! Chronic fatigue is not easy to treat, it takes a lot of patience and perseverance. You are young and strong, and I am sure that now you will have a long, happy and successful life ahead of you!

I would like to draw attention to Catherine's excellent description of her addiction to bread. Grains are addictive, and sugar is considered to be the most addictive substance on the planet. Many people are addicted to these things without realizing it. Our mainstream medicine has no idea of what damage these addictions can do to the health of the person. They can manifest as any chronic disease. In order to heal, it is important for the person to deal with these addictions first.

Catherine Cruchon

Je m'appelle Catherine Cruchon, j'ai 24 ans et voici comment j'ai passé en quelques années du stade de sportive d'élite à celui de ne plus pouvoir me lever de mon lit, pour enfin recommencer à vivre grâce au régime GAPS.

Tout d'abord quelques mots sur ma personnalité : j'ai toujours eu un tempérament un peu hyperactif et perfectionniste. J'essaie d'être la meilleure dans tout ce que j'entreprends. Je ne m'engage par exemple jamais dans une voie où je ne suis pas un minimum douée, car je n'aime pas être derrière. J'ai toujours eu beaucoup d'énergie à dépenser et j'étais fière d'avoir un emploi du temps bien chargé : gymnastique, music, supplément de course à pieds et répétition de music en groupe, puis dès 13 ans trois séances d'aviron par semaine.

À côté de ça, je n'étais que rarement malade. Bien qu'étant plutôt casse-cou et garçon manqué, je ne m'étais jamais cassée quelque chose. J'avais donc confiance en mon corps et me sentais un peu invincible. Mais à bien y réfléchir, les premiers symptômes étaient déjà présents. C'étaient des bouffées de chaleurs qui engendraient des maux de tête. Mon corps gérait mal les changements de température. J'avais, de façon générale, toujours trop chaud. Je n'étais donc pas une adepte des bains de soleil. De toute façon je ne bronzais pas ou peu. Je n'étais pourtant pas sensible au coup de soleil, mais je restais 'blanche'.

J'avais également un sommeil agité. Je me réveillais deux à trois fois par nuit. Toutefois, je me rendormais directement après, si bien que cela ne me gênait pas. Je me souviens avoir eu comme réflexion qu'il fallait simplement que je me dépense physiquement suffisamment tous les jours afin d'arriver à m'endormir.

Plus tard, j'ai déclaré de la dyslexique accompagnée de fort retards de lectures, décrochant ainsi un ticket pour deux heures de logopédie hebdomadaires durant 1 an et demi. Parallèlement, J'ai commencé à faire de l'asthme sous effort et de l'hyperventilation. Ce qui m'a valu une prescription de Ventolin® et de Cortisone.

Durant l'adolescence, je me suis laissée tenter par le chanvre, mais j'ai rapidement constaté que cela ne me convenais pas. Seules deux inhalations de cette fumée m'avaient fait partir en 'bad trip' avec perte de conscience de la réalité, et sensation de dédoublement de moi-même. Cette sensation de perte de contrôle de ma vie m'avait alors suffisamment dégoûtée pour que j'arrête définitivement la cigarette et le cannabis.

En lisant ça on peut se dire que mon enfance était un cauchemar, mais en réalité jusqu'ici tout allait bien. J'avais de la facilité à l'école, je faisais pas mal de sport et me débrouillais bien. J'ai eu quelques problèmes d'intégration avec les autres jeunes de mon âge durant quelques années de mon adolescence, mais à part ça je ne pouvais me plaindre de rien. Mon comportement hyperactif ne m'a jamais gêné, au contraire j'étais fière d'arriver à faire autant de choses tout en réussissant facilement mes études. J'avais de l'énergie et de la motivation toute la journée et j'adorais ça !

J'ai ensuite fait partie de l'équipe nationale Suisse d'aviron. Ma vie se partageait alors entre un travail de vigneronne/caviste à 80% (=métier physique), et 11 séances de 2 heures d'entraînement par semaine, plus 5 semaines de vacances passées en camps d'entraînement où nous avions 2 à 3 entraînements par jour. Ajoutez à cela les sorties avec mes amis dès que l'occasion se présentait. Je me sentais forte et bien dans ma peau. Des amis géniaux, un travail passionnant, et la qualification en poche pour les championnats du monde d'aviron moins de 23 ans.

C'est à 20 ans que les problèmes ont commencés... J'ai alors eu gentiment l'impression de m'endormir. Au début ça me demandait des efforts de marcher après les entraînements, puis ça devenait permanent, je mettais de plus en plus de temps à me changer dans les vestiaires, je n'avais plus d'énergie pour répondre au téléphone en fin de journée, mes résultats à l'entraînement devenaient de moins en moins réguliers. J'ai ensuite commencé à avoir des douleurs dans les membres, c'était une sorte de mal difficile à décrire, quelque chose à l'intérieur, entre le muscle et l'os, un peut comme si mes nerfs étaient compressés. Au final j'avais tellement mal aux jambes et sous les pieds que je n'arrivais plus à marcher. J'avais l'impression d'avoir 300kg qui pesaient sur mes plantes de pieds et des bouts de bois douloureux à la place des jambes.

À côté de cela, je subissais des brûlures d'estomac. Je les ai longtemps confondues avec un sentiment de faim ce qui a perturbé mon alimentation puis mon sommeil. J'avais régulièrement des problèmes de fringale avec des sueurs froides et une sensation de faiblesse alors que j'avais quelque chose dans le ventre. J'avais également beaucoup d'aliments non digérés dans mes celles, spécialement des légumes crus. Je perdais beaucoup mes cheveux qui étaient devenus très fin. J'avais toujours ces bouffées de chaleurs accompagné de transpiration. J'avais souvent de la peine à digérer, je me sentais rarement bien après les repas, j'avais une sensation de pierre dans l'estomac. Lors de repas prolongé j'étais vraiment mal à l'aise à table, il me fallais me lever et me coucher.

Le plus important est que, j'étais hyper fatiguée tout le temps. C'était plus un manque d'énergie et une sensation de faiblesse, qu'un besoin de dormir. Je n'avais simplement plus la force pour rien faire même si je sortais d'une nuit de 12 heures de sommeil.

Au début ces fatigues étaient cycliques, durant 2 à 3 semaines j'étais pleine d'énergie, je pouvais faire la fête constamment jusqu'à point d'heure. J'étais motivée pour tout. Puis, durant un temps équivalent, je dormais sans cesse. Mais à la fin cette fatigue était devenue permanente.

Les brûlures d'estomacs (que je confondais avec la sensation de faim) augmentaient alors gentiment et mes troubles alimentaires avec. Mon corps me demandait de la nourriture comme une toxicomane en manque de drogue. Lorsque j'avais faim, cette sensation occupait ma pensée au point que je me sente rapidement mal sans manger. Il n'y avait que quelques aliments qui pouvaient combler ma faim. C'était principalement du pain, du pain et du pain, ou éventuellement d'autres féculents. Je pouvais manger 300gr de pain pour les 4h et manger normalement pour le souper ensuite. Je mangeais le matin, à midi, à 18h, à 21h à minuit et je devais me relever toutes les nuits vers 4h du matin pour manger quelque chose sans quoi je n'arrivais plus à dormir. Et chaque repas était constitué d'un minimum 150gr de pain ou de céréales sucrées. Il m'était devenu impensable de manger un légume ou un fruit cru sauf éventuellement des bananes ou des avocats. A la fin même boire de l'eau était devenu difficile car j'avais l'impression qu'elle augmentait mes brûlures d'estomac. Je mangeai également beaucoup de produits laitiers ainsi que du sucre sous forme de patte à tartiner au chocolat (3kg en 1 mois) et du beurre de caca-houète à la petite cuillère (400gr/sem voir plus). Je mangeais énormé-ment, car avoir le ventre rempli était la seule chose qui calmait un peu mes brûlures estomac. Du coup j'avais perdu la sensation de satiété. Je mangeais simplement jusqu'à avoir le ventre plein puis j'allais me recoucher. Heureusement pour moi, je ne prends pas facilement du poids car je me faisais peur moi-même en voyant le nombre de calorie journalière que je pouvais avaler !

Paradoxalement, je ressentais tous ces symptômes, mais j'ai mis beaucoup de temps prendre conscience que ce n'était pas normal. C'est comme si j'effaçais ces données de ma tête pour pouvoir continuer mon train de vie. Je mentionnais naturellement à mon médecin que je me sentais fatiguée à chaque fois que j'allais le voir. Il faisait régulièrement des analyses, mais les prises de sangs ne montraient rien d'anormal. Mon médecin minimalisait alors mes propos. Puisqu'il ne s'inquiétait pas, je me persuadais que ce mal n'était que passager. Il y a eu, toutefois, une analyse sanguine qui releva la présence d'une mononucléose terminée. Comme celle-ci a été découverte alors qu'elle n'était déjà plus influente, et que je n'ai ressenti aucune différence entre avant et après, elle ne peut pas constituer une explication à mon problème.

Et c'était pareil pour mes menstruations. Je ne les avais toujours pas trois ans après avoir arrêté le sport. Mais, la encore, mon bilan hormonal ne montrait aucun dérèglement. Des dires de ma gynécologue selon ces analyses, je devais avoir mes règles. Oui mais je ne les avais pas ! Et résultat, je me suis vue prescrire la pilule pour les déclencher...

Au final, j'étais tellement fatiguée et mal qu'il ne fallait pas me demander de calculer 2 + 2, mon cerveau était totalement hors d'usage. Il m'était impossible d'essayer d'organiser quelque chose ou de me projeter dans l'avenir. Par moments j'aurai pu me taper la tête contre les mûres. Sincèrement, heureusement que j'avais encore un brin de raison qui me disait de ne pas péter les plombs parce que, dans le cas contraire, je serai sûrement dans un institut spécialisé à l'heure ou je vous parle.

Je pouvais très bien imaginer que certains enfants finissent autiste, parce que si cela m'étais tombé dessus étant plus jeune, et que je n'aurais donc ma compris ce qui m'arrivait, c'est sûr que j'aurais fini dans un état proche de l'autisme.

C'est seulement lorsque j'ai senti que tout cela me pesait gentiment sur le moral, que j'ai commencé à m'inquiéter sérieusement. Je ne pouvais plus rien faire, je n'avais plus la force d'aller boire un verre avec mes amis. Lors d'une belle journée d'été, je regardais le ciel bleu depuis mon lit en me disant qu'en temps normal j'aurais appelé quelques copains pour aller faire une partie de *beach volley* alors que là j'étais simplement allongée sans avoir la force de ne rien faire. Je n'arrivais même plus à aller travailler. J'avais vraiment l'impression de passer à côté de ma vie et cette situation commençait sérieusement à m'attrister et me peser.

Ma personnalité fait que je n'aurais pas pu passer ma vie à ne rien faire tout en coûtant de l'argent à la société, et cela sans même avoir un nom à mettre sur ce qui n'allait pas chez moi. Je veux dire que si j'avais eu un cancer ou une autre maladie alors là oui, j'aurai pu accepter cette fatigue car j'aurai eu quelque chose contre quoi me battre.

Mais passer ma vie enfermée dans un corps qui ne me laissait rien faire, m'était impossible à concevoir.

Du coup j'ai rappelé mon médecin et cette fois j'étais bien déterminée à trouver ce qu'il n'y allait chez moi ! Parce que si je finissais par faire une dépression, on aurait dit que c'était ça la cause de ma fatigue !

De plus a ce que j'ai pu voir, dès que les médecins ne savent pas trop ce que vous avez, ils vous prescrivent des anti-dépresseurs. Mais je ne voulais surtout pas commencer avec ça car mon passé de sportive m'avait appris à ne pas écouter mon corps et à dépasser mes limites constamment. Ce qui fait que j'avais tendance à ne pas m'arrêter avant d'être dans le rouge. Et avec ma façon de vivre un peu hyperactive j'avais déjà assez de peine à savoir : quand il me fallais lever le pied car j'en faisais trop, quand est ce que j'étais vraiment fatiguée et quand est ce que c'était simplement de la fainéantise de ma part. Alors imaginer prendre des antidépresseurs aurait encore ajouté une couche de confusion à ce qui était déjà pas évident à gérer pour moi.

J'avais alors premièrement eu le droit au diagnostique de surentraînement. J'ai donc gentiment arrêté toute activité physique. Puis ce fût l'hyperactivité. J'ai alors pris la plus forte dose autorisée de rithaline sans vraiment sentir les effets du médicament. Il estompait un peu les bouffées de chaleurs et le sentiment de malaise qui allait avec mais ça ne réglait pas le problème. J'avais en même temps un médicament contre les brûlures d'estomac, qui ne faisait aucun effet. Puis ce fût un médicament contre les jambes impatientes, là encore sans résultat.

Et ce qui me dérangeait le plus c'est que de la gynécologue jusqu'à mon médecin généraliste, je me voyais à chaque fois prescrire une liste de médicaments qui ne faisait que masquer les symptômes sans soigner la cause ! Et je me retrouvais à 24 ans avec 3 médicaments coûteux à prendre par jour sans pour autant me sentir bien.

Un dimanche matin alors que j'étais vraiment à bout car je n'arrivais plus à dormir à cause des brûlures d'estomac et parce que j'en pouvais plus d'être mal à longueur de journée sans solution, je me suis rappelée le régime GAPS dont une amie m'avait parlé et que j'avais très brièvement entamé il y avait de ça deux ans. À ce moment-là, je n'étais pas assez mal pour avoir la motivation d'appliquer ces principes rigoureusement. Mais aujourd'hui j'étais prête à tout.

Et bien croyez-moi ou pas, mais ce fameux dimanche, j'ai arrêté tous médicaments pour commencer à manger selon les principes GAPS et un jour plus tard, je me suis réveillée tellement en forme que je n'y croyais pas moi-même. Bien sûr j'avais encore des brûlures d'estomac ainsi que plusieurs autres choses mais, j'étais pleine d'énergie ! Je me rappelle avoir pu monter les marches d'escaliers deux par deux, avoir des mouvements rapides et un sourire jusqu'aux oreilles à tel point j'avais l'impression de revivre !

J'ai alors repris rendez-vous avec Mme Krüger pour débuter sérieusement, avec son soutien et ces conseils, la diète d'introduction.

La première chose géniale c'est que j'avais enfin une explication qui me paraissais tenir la route sur ce qui n'allait pas chez moi. Puis, J'ai eu comme l'impression d'enfin comprendre mon passé. Le fait de découvrir que tous était lié depuis le fait que je ne bronzais pas ou que mes cheveux étaient devenu si fin, jusqu'à ma fatigue et mes maux de ventre, ma parut soudainement logique.

Le régime ne fût pas facile et j'y suis encore. Imaginez : je suis une œnologue en stage au Etat Unis pour une année et je ne peux pas boire de vins, ni aucun autre alcool. Je ne peux goûter à aucuns des excellents plats qu'apporte chaque jour mes collègues mexicains pour le midi, ou simplement tester les centaines de succulents restaurants de Portland (Oregon). De plus il est beaucoup plus difficile de faire connaissance avec les gens si vous ne pouvez pas partager un apéro, des grillades ou même un café avec eux. Donc non ce n'est pas facile, il faut beaucoup d'organisation pour se procurer tous les aliments indispensables au régime et de planification pour avoir toujours un repas prêt et un frigo rempli. Mais surtout il faut être convaincu des bienfaits du régime car dans le cas contraires il est impossible de ne pas faire d'écarts.

J'avoue ne pas avoir été très strique à mon arrivée: nouveaux horizons, nouveaux amis, week-end camping, BBQ, apéro, café, fêtes... et très vite on se dit : 'allez c'est dans ta tête, je suis sûr que je peux manger juste une tortillas et boire un verre de vin ou une Margarita, ça ira très bien...' Mais en moins de deux semaines, je me suis retrouvée au lit sans avoir la force d'aller travailler...

Je me suis alors reprise en main pour appliquer à la lettre ma diète d'introduction, et comme pas magie, les améliorations reviennent gentiment.

En fait je pense que le plus dur c'est de ne pas pouvoir partager avec les gens qu'on aime. Ce n'est ni la nourriture en elle-même, ni l'alcool ou la caféine qui me manque mais juste l'action de partager un repas ensemble, de boire un verre de vin pour apprécier la fin d'une journée de travail ou une coupe de champagne pour fêter un examen réussi, la glace que l'on mange en se baladant au bord du lac, le brunch entre ami le dimanche matin. C'est définitivement tous ces moments qui me manquent. Mais quand je pense qu'il y a de ça quelques mois j'étais tellement mal et faible que je n'avais même plus la force de marcher, alors qu'aujourd'hui je passe mes journée à parcourir les vignes d'Oregon, je me dit que le jeu en vaut bien la chandelle.

Mais j'espère qu'un jour GAPS sera connu de tous et que le monde de la gastronomie et de la fête sera adapté à nous. Et si j'en crois le nombre de personnes qui après m'avoir questionné me disent que eux aussi ils ont une partie des symptômes GAPS. Je me dis qu'une bonne partie de gens sur cette terre ne pourront plus continuer longtemps à consommer les aliments qui sont produit par la société actuelle sans avoir de plus en plus de problèmes de santé que la médecine classique pourra certainement masquer durant un certain temps mais ne pourra pas guérir.

Pour finir, j'aimerais dire un immense merci à la Doctoresse Campbell-McBride pour ces travaux de recherche ainsi qu'à Mme Krüger-Fantoli pour ses conseilles, à mes parents et à mes soeurs pour leur aide et leur soutien et à mes amis pour leur compréhension !

Sans vous je ne serai pas là aujourd'hui, alors merci du fond du cœur.

21

Marijke de Jong

Key words: Chronic Fatigue Syndrome, back pain, parasites, arthritis, digestive problems

Results of more than two years on GAPS

In 2001 I had an adrenal burnout. I was 57 years old and tired, tired, tired. That is when my search for health started. I learned so much about myself, about gut flora, about possible cures and about food. And in the fall of 2008 I read about the GAPS Nutritional Programme for the first time. I just knew that this was my road to health. I felt it immediately. But when I looked up the details I decided this was not for me. Too difficult! Too weird in my country of bread and potatoes, the Netherlands. So I slowly went low-carb instead.

While on a low-carb diet I started taking Bio-Kult and, to my surprise, I got terribly painful die-off symptoms; then a test showed that my blastocystis was gone. I knew I had this parasite. But the test also showed that I had another single cell parasite: diëntamoeba fragilis. My doctor prescribed an anthroposophical medicine, and after lots of time, back pain and die-off later this parasite left me too. All this made it clear to me that my gut flora was at the root of my problems. So after all I decided to start the GAPS Programme at the end of September 2009, at the age of 65. Being retired I could do all the strange things I wanted. And now, after two years on GAPS, it is a good moment to review my progress. I am not completely healed but I am very much better. At the age of 67 it is to be expected that it takes longer to get rid of all the bad stuff I collected in the years before.

The first year of GAPS was a year of learning. I bought a slow cooker and a juicer. Those two are indispensible now; they are my best GAPS buys. I learned to make bone broth, sauerkraut, yogurt and kefir. I struggled with die-off and learned the lesson to go really slow, though I forget that lesson every so often. I learned to cook pleasant meals for myself. I learned what supplements I needed and they were many. Dr Campbell-McBride prefers us to heal without supplements, but I decided that they were necessary for me. I also learned muscle testing to avoid over-supplementation. I still use that. I learned to cook and eat according to the rules. I somehow managed to eat out now and then.

But, I also cheated. After six months I thought that one slice of bread a day made life a lot easier and would do no harm. I noticed no harm so why bother? But in September, around the one year mark, I suddenly realized that I was not making progress any more. It dawned on me that this programme has to be followed strictly if you want success. So I did and it helped.

In my second year I changed my probiotics strategy. This had a major influence, together with my new faithful adherence to the rules. For a month or two I had waves of die-off every few days. My changing gut flora was now killing off a series of bad invaders. This strengthened my faith in the programme. I redid Intro and expected major improvements. But that did not happen. I felt tired. I felt like I was detoxifying all the time. I stopped honey, fruit and all sweet vegetables. Tried Bio-Kult but could not do it. My liver needed support. My body kept detoxifying heavy metals. And I was still tired, not as much as before, even a lot better than in the beginning, but still tired. So I needed more time.

In the course of the second year things went better and better. I feel now that I have my life back. I make plans for the future and I enjoy myself. Eating GAPS is completely normal for me now. Cookies do not tempt me anymore. I have no wish to go back to my old ways of eating, even when I am completely healed. My blood sugar is steady and I eat three meals a day with no snacks in between. Even skipping lunch is no longer the impossibility it used to be. And now, past the two year mark, the improvement is back to slow and steady.

I am so thankful that I found this programme!

My gains:
I have more energy.
I have a more positive and gentler mood.
My blood sugar is steady.

All my back pains are gone.
Hip and knee pains are gone.
The pain in my foot is gone.
My food sensitivities and growing list of allergies are gone.
I have no more gas rumblings in my belly.
My stool has good consistency where it used to be mushy.
No more stomach cramps or tummy pain.
The sacral-ileal joint (between the spine and the hip bone) that was blocked for years is flexible again.
I have better coordination.
My skin is healthy and firm.
I no longer have smelly armpits or feet.
I do not burn in the sun anymore.
My immune system is strong.
My liver is in good order.
I can lift heavy things.
I plan to keep eating this way and further improve my life.

I am glad I found GAPS and I thank Dr Campbell-McBride for inventing the programme. I hope my story will inspire people to start GAPS, even if they are over 65!

A comment from Dr Natasha

Thank you for sharing your story, Marijke! The human body is an amazing creation: it heals and rejuvenates itself all the time. Just give it the right food and stop polluting it with man-made chemicals, and it will heal on its own without any outside help! And at any age!

22

D.

Key words: chronic fatigue, depression, dental problems, heavy metal toxicity

Hindsight is, of course, always wiser than foresight, they say. 'After the event, even a fool is wise. Yet it is not the hindsight of a fool, but it is the foresight of the reasonable man, which alone can determine responsibility.' (Dieter Giesen, *International Medical Malpractice Law*, page 105). How I wish that my doctors, dentists, family, friends and I had learned in more detail about gut flora/gut dysbiosis and environmental toxins many years ago. Much suffering and probably some untimely death could have been prevented.

When I first read the GAPS book, I both cried and laughed because clear explanations for things which had troubled me for 40+ years jumped off the pages, and so many of the ailments endured by relatives and friends began to slot into the jigsaw puzzle of life, clarifying many matters. Since then, I have reread the *GAPS* and *Put Your Heart in Your Mouth* books and experimented on myself. With GAPS and a combination of the works of Drs Joachim Mutter, Sidney Macdonald Baker and Mark Hyman on mercury, I have achieved mercury/heavy metal and general detoxification to the extent that I now enjoy energy and vitality.

Energy and vitality eluded me for years, as I endured chronic inflammation in my body expressing itself again and again in painful dental troubles; chronic fatigue; depression; 'frozen' and painful joints; worsening eyesight; and a wish to sleep and avoid ever waking up again. I had managed to ease the pain in my joints temporarily through gentle movement in warm showers and, especially, in thermal pools until I could again progress to gentle swimming, Munari mud treatments and other gentle stretching exercises. Perhaps fortunately, my love of life prevented me from walking away into the snow one quiet and dark mid-winter night, never to return. Tempting though the prospect sometimes was, after a walk, I would return home and resolve to live again the next day, relying in such cases on the saying that 'the morning is wiser than the evening'. Relatives and friends would joke that, should I ever momentarily give into the temptation to swim out in the sea to depart from this life in exhaustion, I should be sure to take my passport with me; they were quite confident that, eventually, I would emerge somewhere, perhaps in another country where I would need to identify myself ...Such humour, as well as considerable time spent with horses and dogs, kept me going through some very dark times. If I were to receive just a penny or cent for each day I cried on the way to/from work, because of feeling so exhausted and miserable, I expect quite a considerable sum of money would come together (which would certainly come in handy). On a positive note, I was often – thank God! – fortunate to meet good-hearted strangers who, on the underground or bus would offer me paper handkerchiefs, sweets, smiles and good wishes to cheer me on my way!

That gut flora and nutritional habits are shared within families makes so much sense! Why do so few medical practitioners realize and acknowledge this? As I reflect on my maternal grandparents, it is clear that each of them had gut flora imbalance. My grandfather spent considerable time in the trenches during the First World War, where he was gassed and endured despicable conditions. When he returned to England he suffered nightmares for the rest of his life. When young, he was very athletic and an excellent runner, however – like so many then – he smoked, developed lung cancer and died about a year before I was born. My grandmother had also been very sporty in her youth, however she was known throughout the years for her 'sweet tooth' and was diagnosed with diabetes type two in her seventies, though I suspect that, by then, she had already suffered it undiagnosed for a considerable time.

Their daughter, my mother, suffered from Obsessive Compulsive Disorder and thyroid problems all the years I knew her. She was sure that the treatment she received for her thyroid imbalance only made things worse, and as a not-so-neutral observer I would agree completely. Anyone who has witnessed OCD in a close relative/loved one will understand the anguish for all concerned. My mother could be incredibly kind and thoughtful, but her personality was overshadowed by OCD; her agitated and angry behaviour had a grave impact on our family's life. It was clear to me from a young age that she needed help, and yet the 'help' she was offered by the medical profession was not only unhelpful but actually made things considerably worse. Her diet, which had been frugal and generally healthy until the mid-1950s, deteriorated so that, later, she existed very much on starches and grains. I believe that she, like my siblings and I, was troubled by gluten/gliadin in particular. Her brother/my uncle and his children have also displayed clear signs of gut dysbiosis for as long as I have known them – developing asthma and a number of allergies to food and animals. My father's parents and sibling, conversely, enjoyed robust health and active lives, whilst my father's health was certainly impaired by years of exposure to metals at his place of work, as well as by the stress of my mother's OCD and, I believe, at times by well-intentioned but incorrect advice given to him by medical practitioners.

My mother had four children, of which I am the youngest. My siblings and I led active lives as children, learning to swim and play various team games, to cycle and ride ponies. Each of my siblings has, however, displayed for years what I now understand to be clear signs of gut dysbiosis, gluten/gliadin intolerance and mercury/heavy metal toxic build-up. My oldest brother slid through this toxic burden into obesity, depression/lack of motivation/resignation, heart disease, diabetes, and lung cancer. Chemotherapy, I believe, took his last desire to live. I feel sure that, had we known about GAPS and heavy metal detoxification then, he could be alive today, enjoying his children as they grow up. My second brother has also been debilitated by chronic exhaustion for years. I am delighted that he is now beginning to get back on track with GAPS. My third brother shows clear signs of gut dysbiosis and has not yet reached the point at which he is keen to explore GAPS.

Given that, both in England and in Scotland, I and my schoolmates were put at the mercy of dentists touting amalgam fillings. I can, at 50+, list a great number of school friends who, sadly, have for years suffered the effects of gut dysbiosis and a wide variety of ailments linked to amalgam fillings, dietary choices and, indeed, multiple/unsafe vaccinations and fluoride. Some have already died, whilst others deal now as best they can with lupus, chronic fatigue, depression, tinnitus, 'frozen' and painful limbs, rheumatoid arthritis, obesity, diabetes etc. I am heartened to see that those who implement GAPS and detoxification wholeheartedly achieve significant improvements in their health – often a complete return to good health. How appalling, though, that European 'health' services continue to deny the dramatic role of dental amalgam and gut dysbiosis in promoting diseases such as Alzheimer's, multiple sclerosis, Chronic Fatigue Syndrome, lupus and other autoimmune imbalances.

I am truly grateful to Dr Natasha Campbell-McBride for her work. I am also grateful to the bright kinesiologist, Vera Pfeiffer, who first pinpointed the root causes of my numerous symptoms, which were significantly worsened by the careless and, I believe, irresponsible treatments I received from a succession of, no doubt well-meaning, medical practitioners over the years. These treatments brought me to the lowest point I ever wish to reach when, thoroughly toxic with mercury and other heavy metals, and with a great number of resulting food intolerances, I lost all my hair in a matter of weeks.

It is a little odd to walk around completely bald as a woman, and I smile as I recall what Catherine Aird said: *'If you can't be a good example, then you'll just have to be a horrible warning!'* For years I had been offered antidepressants and antibiotics, though no one was willing (or able) to check for gluten/gliadin, leptin/lectin or lactose intolerance or, indeed, for vitamin D deficiency and gut flora imbalance. Since the root causes of my health problems were found, I have been stonewalled by some people and authorities who, frankly, have a duty to behave better and improve things now and for the future.

To quote Stéphane Hessel, *'It is time for outrage!'* Please support those scientists, experts and medical practitioners who are courageous and ethical enough to tell the truth! Encourage people to implement GAPS and to expect non-toxic, truly nutritious food from food manufacturers, safe (if really necessary) vaccinations from health authorities, support for detoxification and renewed research into non-toxic dental materials, as well as access for all to truly health-promoting treatments from health insurers. Can we please adhere to: *Primum non nocere/Primum nil nocere!* – First, do no harm! – and refrain from poisoning ourselves, one another, animals and our environment with mercury and other toxins!

A comment from Dr Natasha

Thank you for your story, D.! Yes, toxic metals have become a major cause of disease, and our modern dentistry is one of the main sources of mercury toxicity. Many chemicals dentists use in our mouths are toxic, and we swallow them for a long time after the treatment. As these man-made toxins get into the digestive system, they cause damage to the gut flora and the gut wall. Once the gut flora is damaged the person develops GAPS with all the typical symptoms. The good news is that there is a growing number of holistic dentists around the world, who use better practices.

Toxic metals are difficult to remove from the body and it takes a long time to recover afterwards. The GAPS Nutritional Protocol will allow the gut to heal, and very importantly enable your own detoxification system to recover. Once this powerful system starts working, it will remove all sorts of toxins from your body safely, including toxic metals.

23

Emily Jane Butler

Certified GAPS Practitioner

Key words: Crohn's disease, depression, fatigue

Before I heard about the GAPS Program, I had been on The Specific Carbohydrate Diet (SCD) to overcome Crohn's disease, which I had been diagnosed with in childhood. I followed the SCD faithfully for over two years and experienced radical healing results. I was in a new world, learning the power of food as medicine and discovering a renewed pleasure for eating, a joy of cooking, and a passion for holistic health. My 'flare-ups' became a thing of the past, and I was able to avoid further surgery and get off (and stay off!) prescription medications. In fact, doctors told me I no longer had Crohn's disease!

This personal healing journey was so inspiring that I felt called to take my experience and expertise to a new level by going back to school to become a certified, holistic Health Coach. I wanted to show others with gastro-intestinal disorders and autoimmune disease how to heal their body and reclaim their life through the power of nutrition and lifestyle choices. I launched my practice in 2008 and have taken great joy in serving hundreds of people nationwide. Within a few years time, however, I realized that in my personal health I seemed to reach a plateau. Despite all my progress, I still had questions about my health.

I had lingering symptoms. No matter how I tweaked my diet, I could not get rid of those symptoms. While I was grateful to no longer have flare-ups, I still struggled with chronic bloating, gas, constipation and had trouble digesting fats. I was still having some fatigue, hormonal imbalances and adrenal insufficiency too. I started to wonder if I had gone as far as I could go with SCD. I wondered if there could be something more.

I had also recently undergone dental surgery and, like a good patient, I followed my doctor's orders to take a short round of antibiotics, pain killers and nine ibuprophen a day! Needless to say I was in really rough shape after that. My symptoms were all much worse and I was sinking into depression. I knew it was time to go back to the introductory phase of the SCDiet and to seek out 'something more' to help me resolve these symptoms. Fatefully (and gratefully!) my search led me to GAPS!

Being an SCDiet expert already I knew – the dietary principles that GAPS was founded on worked for those with gastrointestinal concerns, and this created an instant relationship of trust. I also knew it was based on sound scientific research from other doctors and nutritional experts, including Dr Sidney Haas, Elaine Gottschall, Dr Weston A. Price and Sally Fallon.

During my health coach training, Sally Fallon was among my favorite teachers. She taught us about the importance of traditional foods in a healthy diet and shared the research of Dr Weston A. Price. He studied how traditional cultures enjoyed good health before they started eating modern processed foods. I found myself beginning to take what I had learned and integrating it into my SCD regimen by eating more home-made broth, soaking nuts and seeds, and starting to experiment with cultured vegetables. I began fantasizing about how great it would be if there was a diet that brought together the best of both the SCD and traditional food worlds. In discovering GAPS, I soon realized that it was in fact my dream-diet come true! GAPS is a beautiful marriage of these two nutritional healing plans of SCD and Nourishing Traditions. It is a thoughtfully designed holistic nutrition and lifestyle programme tailored to help people like me, who struggle with gut-brain related disorders including GI and autoimmune conditions, not only to feel better, but also to reverse illness and to reclaim health.

I started with the GAPS Intro and began experiencing positive changes unfold. I felt the brain fog disappearing and my thinking became more clear. I began to feel calmer and grounded in my body. The abdominal pain was subsiding. My sleep and my mood began improving. My energy started to go up and the bloating started to go down...I knew I was onto something good. As I progressed through the diet, my healing inspired me to begin sharing GAPS with others by teaching GAPS classes and bringing its principles into my health coaching as a new 'power tool' to serve my clients in achieving their health goals.

As my journey into the GAPS world progressed, I found myself continually learning more. I soon realized, this was much more than a diet; it was a holistic lifestyle and, as a health practitioner, I believe a holistic approach is key to healing. We need more than diet alone to heal. I love how Dr Natasha includes guidelines for detoxification, personal care and home products, oral health, environmental health, and how to be well in the increasingly complex modern world in which we live.

While I loved this perspective, integrating it into my life felt over-whelming at times. As a patient I had many questions about whether or not I was 'doing it right' and how to prioritize and interpret the medical information in a way that felt simple and easy to do. As a prac-titioner, I wanted to understand it all more intimately so I could better serve my clients and guide them through their personal healing jour-ney. Then I heard the exciting news about the GAPS Practitioner train-ing program that Dr Natasha was teaching. Needless to say, I enthusiastically jumped on board!

Now, nearly one year after the training, I have continued to inte-grate GAPS wisdom into my healing and lifestyle. The juicing with GAPS shakes has been a delicious treat that has also reduced bloating and improved my overall digestion. The sunbathing has become a renewed ritual that makes me feel alive. The oral health recommenda-tions have brought shining compliments from my dentist.

Along with my personal healing progress, the best part of all is watching my own healing mirrored back to me through serving my clients. I feel so honored to be a witness to their healing and watching it unfold. I enjoy seeing how GAPS is so much more than a dietary approach. It is in fact a beautiful healing art form. It's like a dance of healing with the body and with all of life. It is a journey to self discov-ery that shows us to be our true selves. It teaches us how to slow down, listen, and honor our body's wisdom. It shines a light on our unique gifts and opens us up to the simple life pleasures of good food and good health. It allows us to be our best self, not in spite of our illness, but because of the gems of learning and jewels of discovery that come out of our illness. For this, I am so grateful for the gift of GAPS and to Dr Natasha Campbell McBride for her artfully crafted and skillful work that will bring generations of healing to us and our world.

A comment from Dr Natasha

Thank you very much for your story and your wonderful work! Emily Jane has already helped many people on their healing journey. The lesson we can learn from her story is that the focus is not on what you are NOT eating. The focus should be on what you ARE actually eating on a daily basis! It is not enough to just remove offending foods, but it is essential to eat healing, southing, nourishing foods for breakfast, lunch, dinner and in between.

Emily is right: GAPS is not just a diet, it is a way of life – living WITH Mother Nature rather than in spite of her, working WITH your body rather than throwing things at it. Respecting your body as a wonderful perfect creation, which knows how to heal itself and repair any damage; all we have to do is listen to it and provide the right tools.

24

Michelle

Key words: gluten sensitivity, hormonal problems, premature menopause, osteopenia, allergies

After reading the Gut and Psychology Syndrome by Dr Natasha Campbell-McBride and the GAPS Guide by Baden Lashkov I realized that I have been a GAPS person all of my life. So many things that I have suffered with were described and talked about, and I felt I had definitely found the right path for me. My long distance Health Coach, who is now a GAPS Practitioner, had mentioned the GAPS Diet to me after she had had such great improvement on it. I am so grateful and thankful to her – she has been such an amazing inspiration to me. I have no doubt I would still be stuck where I was before GAPS and possibly feeling even worse. I had told my Health Coach/GAPS Practitioner that I felt better on GAPS in six months than I felt on the Specific Carbohydrate Diet (SCD) after two and a half years. I remember, after my first GAPS meal with just bone stock and chicken I felt so nourished and satisfied. I honestly don't think I had ever felt that way before after eating. It was a wonderful feeling. My stomach had never been so flat. It has always been bloated and, since starting with severe digestive problems in 2007, it started feeling hard and painful as well. I thought having lots of painful gas and feeling tired was normal.

I was diagnosed as gluten sensitive in January 2008; after going gluten-free I initially felt much better, but gradually my symptoms came back and I started the Specific Carbohydrate Diet in September 2008. I felt great relief from my joint pain, fatigue and brain fog after starting the SCD. I believe I was so toxic that even a little of the bone broth caused severe die-off and I could tolerate very few vegetables. I had to stop fruit for a long time also. I had to go really slowly in introducing foods and was able to introduce very few things during those two and a half years. I do believe though, that eating the few things I could tolerate on SCD and never eating any illegals helped to prepare my body for the GAPS diet. I have been on the GAPS Introduction diet since June 2011 (one year), I'm on stage five and feeling better and better each day. I'm able to move a little quicker with increasing my probiotics and fermented foods recently, and that is helping a great deal. The die-off is becoming less with each increase and I feel myself getting stronger. I am so thankful to have found a local GAPS Practitioner in my area, when Dr Natasha listed them on her website at the end of last year. I have been working with her and she has helped me so much in the last three months.

I have had many health issues since I was a child that included: bed wetting, allergies (I was sick at least twice a year in the Spring and Fall), yeast infections in my 20's, cervical dysplasia, osteopenia at the age 36, low estrogen and progesterone at the age 36 causing all sorts of menopausal symptoms, premature ovarian failure diagnosed at the age 39, large polyp on my colon, gluten sensitivity, toxoplasmosis parasite, and breast cysts.

I am so thankful to Dr Natasha Campbell-McBride. She is truly sent from heaven. I am also very thankful for my two wonderful GAPS Practitioners that I have been working with. I never thought I'd be feeling this good! I still have a long way to go, but I have come a long way. It's a very slow journey for me but has been so worth it. At times it was a little hard to believe those who had been through it, who kept saying to just hang in there and stick with it. But I did, and I can honestly say that I totally understand now what they meant. I can feel each day my body getting closer and closer to completely healing, and I feel so blessed. I'm so very thankful that I'm getting my life back!

A comment from Dr Natasha

Thank you for your story, Michelle! Working with a Certified GAPS Practitioner can make all the difference in the world! These people are not only good professionals, but most of them went through their own health challenges and have invaluable first-hand experience in healing. They have patience and compassion, because they know what it is like trying to recover from chronic illness. You will find a GAPS Practitioner close to you on www.gaps.me.

25

Maria

Key words: narcolepsy, cataplexy attacks, depression

I was diagnosed with Narcolepsy (with frequent Cataplexy attacks) at the age of 17. For the first few years the narcolepsy was controlled relatively well with medication, but by the age of 38 I was a complete wreck, extremely overweight, depressed, falling, dropping things, and sleeping about 17 hours out of 24. Then a friend recommended I read your book ...

From the first full day on the GAPS diet I've had no day-time sleeping, no cataplexy attacks, no depression. I've stopped all my medication and feel better than I've done for years. I've also lost 9lb in the eight weeks I've been on the diet. My family can hardly believe the change! My husband and children are also sticking to the diet and feeling really well.

Of course, I've a long way to go yet, lots of candida to get rid of, but now I know I can do it, and I know how to do it, thanks to you. My family and friends are all so amazed at the amount of energy I have now, and many of them are trying GAPS for themselves.

I am writing to ask you to consider adding 'Narcolepsy' to the list of problems you can help on your website. I went back to the sleep specialist I've been attending in Dublin, hoping she might tell other patients about GAPS but she refuses to believe the improvement had anything to do with the diet! I don't want any publicity for myself but I hate to think of people suffering needlessly. I've always been told that there's no cure for narcolepsy but THERE IS! GAPS!

Thank you for writing *Gut and Psychology Syndrome*!

A comment from Dr Natasha

Yet another mental problem helped by GAPS Nutiritonal Protocol. Our human brain is a physical organ; it needs feeding all the time (and it is a very hungry organ, sponging up at least 25% of all nutrients from your blood), and it needs to be clean (allowed to function without toxicity bombarding it). Nutrition comes out of your digestive system, and 99% of anything toxic in your blood also comes out of your digestive system. So, with any and every mental problem, before trying anything else (medication in particular), attend to your brain's needs by feeding it well and lifting the toxic 'fog' off it. GAPS Nutritional Protocol will do both for you.

Thank you very much for your story, Maria!

Index

Addictions 24–40, 107–114,
    120–124, 189–195, 199–205,
    206–210, 232–243
ADHD (Attention Deficit
    Hyperactivity Disorder)
    61–66, 90–94, 120–124,
    127–134, 232–243
Adopted children 67–75, 107–114
Alcohol abuse 189–195, 199–205
Allergies 3–8, 46–48, 52–54, 95–99,
    115–119, 120–124, 127–134,
    135–148, 183–188, 199–205,
    220–223, 256–258
Amenorrhoea 232–243
Anaemia 157–160, 161–165,
    175–180
Anorexia 24–40, 199–205
Antibiotics, overuse 76–78, 79–81,
    100–106, 120–124, 135–148,
    172–174, 199–205
Anxiety 61–66, 95–99, 135–148,
    157–160, 172–174, 183–188,
    199–205, 206–210, 211–215,
    220–223, 229–231
Apathy 211–215
Arthritis 157–160, 181–182,
    217–219, 220–223, 244–246,
    247–251
Asthma 90–94, 95–99, 115–119,
    127–134, 183–188, 199–205,
    220–223, 232–243
Autism 9–17, 18–23, 55–57, 58–60,
    61–66, 67–75, 79–81, 82–83,

84–89, 95–99, 107–114,
    115–119, 127–134, 149–155
Autoimmunity 41–45, 127–134,
    206–210

Back pain 220–223, 244–246
Bipolar disorder (manic-depressive
    disorder) 100–106, 196–198
Blood sugar instability 120–124,
    199–205, 206–210, 220–223,
    232–243

Candida 49–51, 90–94, 120–124,
    232–243
Cataplexy 259
Celiac disease 189–195, 199–205
Chest pain 95–99
Cholesterol and lipids, elevated
    175–180
CFS (Chronic Fatigue Syndrome)
    49–51, 52–54, 90–94,
    127–134, 232–243, 244–246
Colitis 161–165, 169–171,
    181–182, 252–255
Constipation 3–8, 61–66, 90–94,
    95–99, 127–134, 189–195,
    199–205
Crohn's disease 161–165, 252–255
Cyclical vomiting syndrome
    95–99, 183–188
Cystitis 175–180

Dental problems 247–251

261

Depersonalisation Syndrome (DP)
    211–215
Depression 52–54, 95–99,
    115–119, 127–134, 157–160,
    189–195, 196–198, 199–205,
    206–210, 211–215, 216,
    220–223, 224–226, 247–251,
    252–255, 259
Diarrhoea 90–94, 161–165,
    181–182, 224–226
Digestive disorders 3–8, 61–66,
    67–75, 90–94, 95–99,
    115–119, 120–124, 127–134,
    135–148,166–168, 172–174,
    175–180, 181–182, 183–188,
    189–195, 199–205, 206–210,
    232–243, 244–246, 252–255,
    256–258
Dravet syndrome (a form of
    epilepsy) 76–78
Drugs, long-term use 120–124,
    135–148, 181–182, 199–205,
    220–223, 232–243
Drug abuse 189–195, 199–205
Dyslexia 232–243

Ear infections 3–8, 55–57, 61–66,
    67–75, 79–81, 100–106
Eating disorder 24–40, 120–124,
    199–205
Eczema 46–48, 58–60, 61–66,
    90–94, 115–119, 127–134,
    135–148, 149–155, 206–210
Endometriosis 157–160
Epilepsy 67–75, 76–78
Eye problems 227–228,
    247–251

Failure to thrive 49–51, 127–134
Fatigue 52–54, 61–66, 67–75,
    90–94, 127–134, 157–160,
    183–188, 196–198, 199–205,
    211–215, 220–223, 224–226,

    232–243, 244–246, 247–251,
    252–255
Food intolerances 3–8, 46–48,
    49–51, 84–89, 127–134,
    135–148, 175–180, 199–205,
    244–246, 247–251
Food poisoning 166–168
FPIES (Food Protein Induced
    Enterocolitis Syndrome)
    46–48
Fussy eater 9–17, 18–23, 24–40,
    79–81, 84–89, 120–124

GERD (Gastro Esophageal Reflux
    Disease) 135–148, 232–243
Gluten sensitivity 256–258

Hay fever 127–134, 183–188,
    220–223
Hair loss 127–134, 232–243,
    247–251
Headaches 52–54, 61–66, 67–75,
    115–119, 120–124, 183–188,
    199–205, 232–243
Heavy metal toxicity 247–251
Heart problems 41–45, 157–160,
    229–231
Homocysteine, elevated 175–180
Hyperactivity 61–66, 67–75,
    90–94, 120–124, 127–134,
    232–243

IBS (Irritable Bowel Syndrome)
    157–160, 224–226
Immune system insufficiency 3–8,
    49–51, 90–94, 115–119,
    120–124, 135–148, 157–160,
    211–215, 183–188
Infertility 157–160

Joint pain 95–99, 127–134,
    199–205, 220–223, 224–226,
    244–246, 247–251

Kawasaki disease 3–8
Kidney reflux 76–78

Lead poisoning 84–89
Lupus 127–134

Malabsorption / malnourishment /
   low weight & poor growth
   41–45, 52–54, 90–94,
   115–119, 157–160, 172–174,
   175–180
ME (Myalgic Encephalomyelitis)
   49–51, 90–94
Memory problems 224–226
Menopause 229–231, 244–246,
   256–258
Menstrual problems 120–124,
   183–188, 199–205, 211–215,
   232–243
Mental 'fog' 172–174, 199–205,
   224–226, 232–243
Mental illness 115–119, 120–124,
   183–188, 189–195, 196–198,
   199–205, 206–210, 211–215
Metal toxicity 247–251
Migraines 115–119, 183–188,
   199–205
Milk allergy 52–54, 58–60, 61–66,
   206–210, 220–223
Milk raw 169–171
Miscarriage 157–160
Mitral valve prolapse (MVP)
   229–231
Mold, moldy building 183–188
Mood problems 52–54, 67–75,
   120–124, 127–134, 183–188,
   220–223

Narcolepsy 259
Neurological problems 41–45,
   224–226, 227–228
Neuropathy 224–226, 227–228
Night terrors 58–60

Obesity 199–205
Obsessions 67–75, 120–124,
   199–205
OCD (Obsessive–Compulsive
   Disorder) 95–99, 120–124,
   125–126, 135–148, 199–205
ODD (Oppositional–Defiant
   Disorder) 95–99, 120–124,
   127–134
Osteopenia 256–258

PANDAS (Pediatric Autoimmune
   Neuropsychiatric Disorders
   Associated with Streptococcal
   infections) 125–126,
   127–134, 135–148
Panic attacks 183–188
PANS (Pediatric Acute-Onset
   Neuropsychiatric Syndrome)
   135–148
Parasites 244–246
PCOS (Polycystic Ovaries
   Syndrome) 199–205
PDD-NOS (Pervasive
   Developmental Disorder –
   Not Otherwise Specified)
   79–81, 84–89, 149–155
Plantar fasciitis/painful feet
   220–223, 227–228
PMS (Peri-Menstrual Syndrome)
   120–124, 157–160, 199–205,
   220–223
Postnatal depression 157–160
Probiotics 125–126
Psoriasis 217–219
Psoriatic arthritis 217–219

Reflux 3–8, 67–75, 95–99,
   135–148, 232–243
Restless legs syndrome 232–243
Rosacea 206–210

Schizophrenia 107–114

Seizures 67–75, 76–78
Sensitivity to molds, chemicals and
    EMF (electro-magnetic fields)
    183–188
Sensitivity to noise 224–226
Sinusitis 175–180, 206–210,
    220–223
Sleep apnea 224–226
Sleeping problems 120–124,
    157–160, 172–174, 199–205,
    220–223, 224–226, 232–243
Stamina, poor 211–215, 224–226,
    232–243
Stress, intolerance and damage
    from 157–160, 175–180,
    183–188, 206–210
Sugar craving / addiction 41–45,
    95–99, 107–114, 120–124,
    199–205, 206–210, 220–223,
    232–243
Suicide attempt 199–205

Tantrums 3–8, 61–66, 120–124,
    127–134

Thyroid problems 41–45,
    175–180, 232–243
Tics 135–148
Twins 84–89

Ulcerative colitis 161–165,
    169–171
Urinary problems 67–75, 135–148,
    175–180, 199–205

Vaccine damage 127–134, 135–148
Vaginal thrush 120–124, 157–160,
    199–205
Vegetarian, vegan 24–40, 157–160,
    199–205, 211–215
Vomiting, cyclical vomiting
    syndrome 95–99, 183–188,
    199–205

Weight, excessive 135–148,
    199–205, 220–223

Yeast/fungal infection 120–124,
    183–188, 199–205